QIGONG FOR STAYING YOUNG

"While many books on qigong describe general practices, Qigong for Staying Young *is written by an acupuncturist with many years clinical experience, and gives practical applications that people can do for themselves for a wide range of common conditions. We will be wholeheartedly recommending this invaluable book to our students and patients for many years to come.*"

JAMES MACRITCHIE AND DAMARIS JARBOUX,
FOUNDING BOARD MEMBERS OF THE NATIONAL QIGONG (CHI KUNG) ASSOCIATION USA, CO-
DIRECTORS OF THE CHI KUNG SCHOOL AT THE BODY-ENERGY CENTER, BOULDER, COLORADO,
AND AUTHORS OF *CHI KUNG—ENERGY FOR LIFE*

"*Bravo! What a wonderful, in-depth, and heartfelt offering this book is. Shoshanna has certainly honored her teachers in sharing the practical and rich wisdom flowing in these pages. It is a gift to women of all ages, a tool for life. The healing benefits that come from sincere Qigong practice can truly be sampled in Shoshanna's fine work.*"

FRANCESCO GARRI GARRIPOLI,
PRODUCER OF THE PBS TELEVISION DOCUMENTARY *QIGONG: ANCIENT CHINESE HEALING FOR
THE TWENTY-FIRST CENTURY*, AUTHOR OF *QIGONG: ESSENCE OF THE HEALING DANCE*, AND
CHAIRMAN OF THE NATIONAL QIGONG ASSOCIATION AND **DAISY LEE-GARRIPOLI**, LMT,
WRITER, QIGONG INSTRUCTOR, AND MARTIAL ARTS PRACTITIONER

"*I'm so glad to see another learned female qigong practitioner bringing qigong information and experience to Americans. Qigong has been practically effective for holistic health care for thousands of years. It is a lifelong tool for preserving health, safely and cheaply. This is the value Shoshanna offers to her readers.*"

YANLING JOHNSON,
VICE PRESIDENT OF THE QIGONG ASSOCIATION OF AMERICA AND AUTHOR OF *A WOMAN'S
QIGONG GUIDE; QIGONG FOR LIVING; QI, THE TREASURE & POWER OF YOUR BODY;* AND *QI ENERGY
IN FOODS FOR LIVING*

"*This magnificent work is an incredible distillation of an enormous body of knowledge, and yet it is so readable and clear.* Qigong for Staying Young *will be welcomed by newcomers to qigong as well as seasoned practitioners.*"

MARCIA WEXLER KERWIT, M.P.H, PH.D.,
SENIOR INSTRUCTOR OF HEALING TAO AND DIRECTOR OF BAY AREA HEALING TAO,
CO-AUTHOR OF *HEALING LOVE THROUGH THE TAO* AND *MENOPAUSE MYTHS & FACTS*

"*In her new book,* Qigong for Staying Young, *Shoshanna Katzman has provided a deep instruction not only on qigong exercise, but on the deep and profound benefits qigong has to offer the modern world and particularly the modern woman. Shoshanna has given the world of qigong and the world at large a great gift in this book. My advice? READ IT!*"

BILL DOUGLAS,
FOUNDER OF THE WORLD T'AI CHI & QIGONG DAY, PRESENTER OF THE DVD SERIES
ANTHOLOGY OF T'AI CHI & QIGONG: THE PRESCRIPTION FOR THE FUTURE, AND AUTHOR OF *THE
COMPLETE IDIOT'S GUIDE TO T'AI CHI & QIGONG*

"*Shoshanna explains what many Chinese keep secret: the special needs of women, and exactly how each movement activates the qi flow essential to radiant health. A must-have for anyone interested in taking control of their own health.*"

MICHAEL WINN,
PAST PRESIDENT OF THE NATIONAL QIGONG ASSOCIATION AND FOUNDER OF THE HEALING
TAO USA RETREATS AND CO-WRITER OF SEVEN BOOKS WITH MANTAK CHIA

"Qigong for Staying Young *is an empowering workbook showing women of all ages how to obtain great health benefits from ancient breathing exercises. Practicing the exercises in this book daily can renew your vitality and boost the quality of your life.*"

MICHAEL REED GACH, PH.D.,
AUTHOR OF *ACUPRESSURE'S POTENT POINTS*

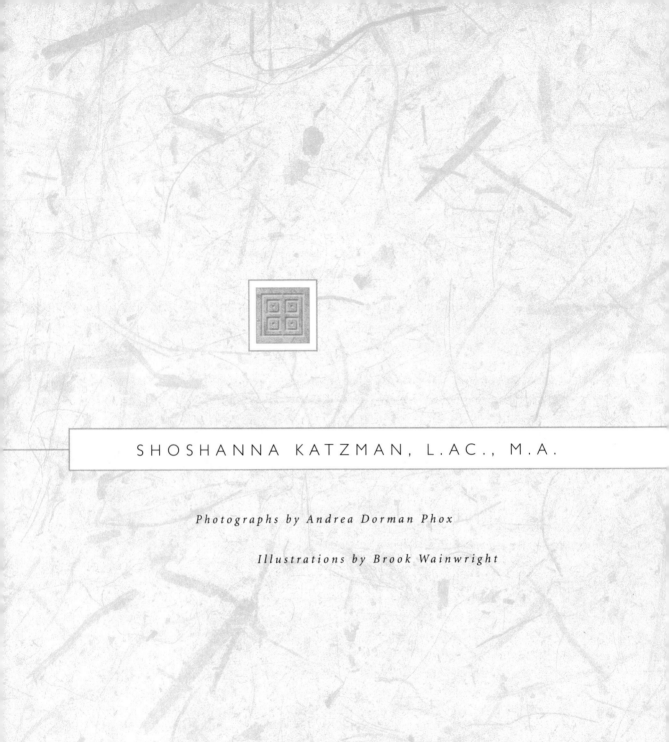

SHOSHANNA KATZMAN, L.AC., M.A.

Photographs by Andrea Dorman Phox

Illustrations by Brook Wainwright

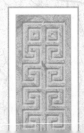

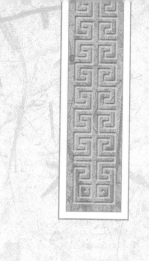

QIGONG FOR STAYING YOUNG

*A Simple Twenty-Minute Workout
to Cultivate Your Vital Energy*

AVERY · A MEMBER OF PENGUIN GROUP (USA) INC. · NEW YORK

AVERY

a member of
Penguin Group (USA) Inc.
375 Hudson Street
New York, NY 10014
www.penguin.com

Library of Congress Cataloging-in-Publication Data

Katzman, Shoshanna.
    Qigong for staying young : a simple 20-minute workout to cultivate
your vital energy / Shoshanna Katzman.
        p.   cm.
    ISBN 1-58333-173-5 (alk. paper)
    1. Qi gong—Health aspects.   2. Physical fitness.   I. Title.
RA781.8.K38   2003   2003050243
613.7'1—dc21

Printed in the United States of America
10   9   8   7   6   5   4   3   2   1

This book is printed on acid-free paper. ∞

BOOK DESIGN BY TANYA MAIBORODA

Acknowledgments

MANY thanks to all those who have guided me throughout my qigong career, especially to my illustrious tai chi, kung fu, and qigong teachers, Bing Gong, Fong Ha, and Larry Johnson. Your faith in me and your love for the internal arts has sustained my practice. Thanks, too, to my students, whose joy in learning and many questions have taught me to be a better teacher.

A special thanks to my Chinese medicine tutors Michael Tierra and Miriam Lee, and instructors Ted Kaptchuk, Subhuti Dharmananda, and Mark Seem, and the Tri State College of Acupuncture faculty, whose combined efforts have imbued me with the ancient knowledge of acupuncture, acupressure, dietary therapy, and herbal medicine.

I would also like to acknowledge my dear teacher Christine Schenk, who has shown me how to blossom as a whole being. Many of the energetic insights shared in this book have come from the energy body therapy I learned from Christine.

There are several other qigong and Oriental medicine instructors who have had an impact on my abilities through intensive workshops. They are Stephen Birch, Luke Chan, Roger Jahnke, Angela Longo, Kiiko Matsumoto, Chulin Sun, Yun Xiang Tseng, Stuart Watts, Frank Yurasek, and Lonny Jarrett. I would also like to thank Ken Cohen for his video *Qigong: Traditional Chinese Exercises for Healing Body, Mind, and Spirit*, on which I based some exercises in set 2.

I have been blessed with so much assistance in bringing this book to fruition. It would not have been possible without the following people:

Kyra Ryan's substantial contributions and commitment to writing excellence gave direction to my creative process. Winifred Golden from Castiglia Agency gifted me with her confidence and the creation of a wonderful connection with my publisher. These two women have been the cornerstones of this project from the very beginning. I would never have had the pleasure and good fortune of knowing Kyra and Winifred if it weren't for my dear childhood friend Steven Schwartz, whose highly spirited and talented friend, Liza Nelligan, brought us together.

A special thank-you to Kristen Jennings at Avery for being a fabulous editor and for her creative flare in shaping the book's final form. And to Laura Shepherd, my appreciation for acquiring the book and for believing in my potential.

Many thanks and appreciation for the hours and love devoted to this project from Andrea Dorman Phox. Andrea's keen ability to look through the eye of a camera and capture the art of reality amazes me—what a talent! Brook Wainwright did an incredible job of blending medical illustration and Chinese medicine through the artistry of her hand. Both Andrea and Brook have brought beauty, professionalism and a woman's touch to this book.

I have been so moved by the generosity and support of Adrian Rodriguez of Elizabeth Arden's Red Door Salon in New York, who gave up precious Sundays with his daughter to be with me for photo shoots. Not only did Adrian give me a great "do" but his unique flare and vision helped mine immensely.

Thank you to Melissa Adams for makeup artistry. Shannon Mincieli for calming direction, and Jill Garfunkel for culinary delights during our arduous shoots. Many thanks go out to Mike and Bill at Monmouth Camera for their "over and above" dedication to helping Andrea create the best photos possible.

I so appreciate the time and energy given by Kimberly Carroll, who has kept my acupuncture center together and spent hours helping me edit the manuscript during the long days and nights leading up to submission. Thanks for holding my hand, literally, through those hours. To Steve Lowy and Malvin Finkelstein for all the time reviewing the manuscript and giving it their stamps of approval, many thanks.

Thank you also to my dedicated staff and patients at Red Bank Acupuncture, my qi sisters and brothers from the National Qigong Association, and my dear friends and family—my beloved parents, five sisters, and many in-laws—for your love and support.

Last but by no means least, many heartfelt thanks to my husband, Michael, who brought his Internet expertise and organizational support to the project, in addition to keeping me fed, caring for our children, and creating the space for me to flourish. And to my children, Hilary, Noah, and Jared who have shared their mommy with her "book baby" for more hours than they would have chosen, thank you. I so enjoyed those special moments of writing together, in tandem, on our computers!

This book is dedicated to my Mom-Mom Wachs and Bubbie Seidman,
and to the grandmothers and great-grandmothers of all time.

Contents

Foreword

IT IS ESTIMATED that worldwide 200 million people practice qigong (Chinese yoga) or tai chi every day—a number nearly equal to that of the entire population of the United States. What would happen if that many Americans sincerely optimized both health and inner peace every day? It would end the health-care crisis and save approximately a trillion dollars that is currently spent—some would say wasted—on medical services for diseases that are preventable or doctor visits that are not needed.

In addition to having the power to cure their own diseases and save the nation billions of dollars, individuals who practice qigong and tai chi (or the sister practice from India, yoga) can have more energy, maintain their youth, think more clearly, decrease stress, access inner peace, get more done, and have more fun. This is a promise worth pursuing given that the cost of participating is nothing.

I am sincerely honored to have the opportunity to introduce this comprehensive, timely, and inspiring book by Shoshanna Katzman. *Qigong for Staying Young* will become an instant classic in the emerging Western literature on qi, qigong, tai chi, and the Chinese healing arts. This book creates a powerful entry point for a whole new wave of women as well as men who will begin practicing qigong and become empowered to be the solution to their own challenges—and it will help reinstate self-reliance in our culture.

For those with background in tai chi, qigong, or yoga, *Qigong for Staying Young* will further inform, inspire, and deepen their understanding of their practice. This book will affect the health-care system, and also schools, social service agencies, community centers, churches, and businesses because caring for health doesn't just happen in hospitals, doctors' offices, and pharmacies. Caring for health happens at home, at work, at school, and in faith communities. *Qigong for Staying Young* will be used in all of these contexts as well as in spas and retreats.

How do people like Shoshanna (who is from New Jersey) and myself (originally from Ohio and now California) become immersed in the physical, mental, and spiritual traditions of ancient China? One reason looms large— energy and power, the qi. We love vitality, self-reliance, and inner peace; in China these are intimately linked with the qi.

The Chinese figured out, millennia ago, what we in the West are just beginning to explore: the concept that you can decide to maximize yourself by cultivating the qi. This is like a wonder of the world; we may eventually find that it is one of the major breakthroughs of the twenty-first century, fully 5,000 years after the Chinese first discovered qi.

Ancient Chinese tradition is gifting the Western world with some amazing breakthroughs: healing can be applied before you are sick to optimize health; profound healing resources are produced naturally within the human body for free; health care is not limited to medications and surgical procedures, rather it is a way of life, a way of being; and there are practical approaches to both aging and agelessness. This gift will transform both our medicine and our culture.

I remember meeting Shoshanna for the first time at a workshop I presented at the annual conference of the American Association of Acupuncture and Oriental Medicine. Before we started, she was off to the side doing a lovely qigong form. I remember thinking to myself that she was obviously adept and that she was involved deeply enough to use spare time to return to her practice. Later, during a sharing session we were discussing how qigong would affect America and she made some remarks that suggested to me that she would be a likely person to spread the good news of qigong. I remember very clearly predicting, "Don't be surprised if you one day create a set of qigong practices, based in your knowledge, personal experience, and enthusiasm."

Now, here it is—a practical, eloquent set of practices founded in Chinese medicine, that Shoshanna has created from traditional sources with great care and attention—for you. Her many years of experience as an acupuncturist, tai chi and qigong practitioner and teacher are woven together with her insights from the feminine, creating a wealth of knowledge and wisdom on accessing and sustaining health in your body, mind, and spirit.

The original medicine of all ancient cultures was primarily developed by the grandmothers. My own first and favorite master teacher of both Chinese medicine and qigong is a woman. When qigong and tai chi are used as tools toward balance and harmony, they potentiate us all—women and men. The flowing movements, the gentle power and the grace of qigong and tai chi support women in harnessing their inner power of strength and surrender. Through the practice men also cultivate the inner power of strength and surrender.

This book, while it speaks eloquently to women, taps a body of knowledge that in no way is limited to gender, age group, level of intellect, or sector of society. Qi cultivation is a power tool, accessible to everyone who aspires to maximize for their own good and the good of others and *Qigong for Staying Young* is an excellent revelation of that deep and wide body of knowledge.

You are standing at a gateway to an amazing world of practical wonder. Why do a reported 100 million people in China go into the parks in the very early morning to practice their physical, mental, and spiritual fitness routines? In the winter in Beijing it is cold and it is dark, and yet they are there. This is immensely intriguing.

Standing at this gateway, holding this book in your hands you are either already practicing or you are considering practicing qigong or tai chi. In either case you are holding a key to inspired living and personal transformation.

Roger Jahnke, O.M.D.
Author, *The Healer Within* and *The Healing Promise of Qi*
April 2003
Santa Barbara, California
Institute of Integral Qigong and Tai Chi
http://FeeltheQi.com

If the Spirit receives proper nourishment,
there is nothing that will not grow.
If it loses proper nourishment,
there is nothing that will not decay.

MENG TZU,
THE WORKS OF MENCIUS

The real trick is to stay alive as long as you live.

ANN LANDERS

Introduction: *Becoming Ageless*

WHAT IS QIGONG?

The word *qigong* (pronounced "chee-gung") is derived from two Chinese characters. The first, *qi* (or chi), refers to our vital energy, life force, or breath. It is the energy that pulses through all living things, the force that passes between you and your loved ones, or the spark that allows you to turn a good idea into an action. Sometimes translated as "the vapor of the finest matter," the Chinese character for qi represents the steam that rises from a grain of cooking rice, symbolizing distilled essence. The second character, *gong*, means "practice" or "cultivation." Qigong, then, is the cultivation of the vital energy the Chinese call qi, the force that animates every living being.

Practicing the art of qigong opens the flow of qi not only in the area we are moving but throughout our bodies. When balanced and strengthened by qigong practice, our qi keeps us fit and healthy all our lives.

Though qigong has been studied by physicians of traditional Chinese medicine for thousands of years, Western scientists in both China and the

United States have only recently begun to apply scientific method to the practice. Initial studies of qigong and the related qi-cultivating exercise tai chi show that regular practice lowers blood pressure; improves heart function; eases addictions; significantly reduces falls and fractures in the elderly; and reduces fatigue, anxiety, tension, depression, and mental confusion at any age. Qigong has been popularly associated with astounding acts by masters who move objects just by pointing their fingers, illuminate lightbulbs merely by holding them in their hands, or dissolve tumors without even touching a patient's body. Enthusiasts believe that the practice cures a variety of illnesses from heart disease to arthritis, asthma to AIDS. Though recent studies aim to measure qi via bioluminescent imagery or to chart the effects of qigong on illness, the vital force of qi has yet to be fully grasped with conventional methods.

Given the growing popularity of Eastern medicine in our country, it is likely that by the time Western science is finally able to chart and describe all that qi does, millions of Americans will have already experienced the power of this vital energy.

Of the four major branches of traditional Chinese medicine—acupuncture, herbal medicine, qigong, and massage—qigong is the most easy to practice as a self-healing technique. With the exception of external or medical qigong, which relies on a practitioner who emits qi and moves it through your body, no one else can do qigong for you. All you need is your own qi! When you practice qigong, you perform a set of graceful movements and postures that are like a simple dance, one designed to balance the vital energy throughout your body. The practice also includes meditation and visualization, self-massage, and the expression of sounds. When you practice qigong regularly, your health and fitness are in your very own hands. Subtle yet powerful, the results of your practice will astound you.

QIGONG AND THE AGELESS WOMAN

In ancient China, in the time before the dynasties of kings, it is said that healers were mature women, shamans with magical powers who came from the South. In fact, one of the original meanings of the ideogram for woman, *wu*, may have been "to heal." Since the practice of qigong originated during this era of women healers (prior to 500 B.C.), it is likely that older women were deeply involved in the inception of the art of cultivating qi. This would explain why, in addition to its many other benefits, qigong is so well suited to the mature woman's needs.

In traditional Chinese medicine, it is believed that good health is achieved when there is a balance of yin and yang, the polar opposites that comprise every part of the natural world. Every human being is made up of a combination of yin and yang. Men's energy is seen to be more yang—outwardly focused, hard, hot, and dry—while women are typically more yin—inward looking, soft, cold, and wet. Whatever our natural individual tendencies, the goal of qigong practice for women is generally to balance our yin and yang. Building yang warms us, strengthens our blood, sparks our sexual energy, and even helps us to speak our minds and access a certain hard edge when necessary. On the other hand, when our yin is depleted, as it often can be when we juggle a multitude of demands, including career and family, qigong helps us to nourish it. This helps us to soften and go inward, drawing on our natural feminine power. Because it balances emotions, promotes serenity, and strengthens the body, qigong is key to healthful longevity. Qigong is a gentle, slow, life-enhancing form of exercise that can be practiced anywhere by anyone. The workout I have designed is specially tailored for women over thirty-five.

After thirty-five, there is no denying that our bodies change. Our skin can become less resilient, headaches and body aches may be more common, and hair and bones can become more brittle. These physical changes, an increase in chronic pain, and the onset of menopause can sometimes lead to depression and despair. Our hormones are changing, and we may experience low energy and a decline in our sexual drive. Hardly what we wish for in what are supposed to be our golden years! But when we diligently perform qigong, our body's aging process can be greatly reduced, even reversed. When we embrace the ancient practice of qigong, our thirty-five-plus years become the most vibrant, vital time of our lives. The power of qi is amazing indeed, and when we learn to harness it, we flower into the sexy, powerful, vital mature women we were born to be. Qigong tones the mind, body, and spirit. Its results can seem miraculous.

Besides its many physical benefits, practicing qigong for just a short time on a daily basis gives you the fortitude to concentrate on your goals and achieve them. It develops your intuition and promotes peace of mind. It brightens your smile, helping you to look and feel younger, more graceful, and even more hopeful.

So, if you are like many of the women I see in my acupuncture practice, you want to avoid depression, sickness, and debility in the latter part of your life. Perhaps you want to heal from an existing disease and attain a better quality of life. If are you ready to stop doing everything for everyone besides yourself, ready to nurture your mind, body, and spirit on a profound new level, this exercise form is for you. Devote just twenty minutes to the gentle practice of qigong and you will create longevity, shining health, enjoyment, and vital energy for yourself in what can truly be your golden years.

HOW TO USE THIS BOOK

Not just a physical exercise, qigong is an alternative/complementary form of medicine with numerous health benefits including detoxification and strengthening of all the organ functions in the body. More and more physicians recommend qigong because it is so gentle. However, it should not be used as a substitute for medical treatment without first consulting your physician. It is suitable for people of all ages and physical abilities, especially older people and those recovering from illness or injury. When you practice qigong, do so at your own pace, respecting your own special needs and limitations.

In the pages that follow, I have synthesized my studies and experience with the wide world of Chinese medicine to bring you a simple, practical plan to help you look and feel younger. With its Eastern concepts (qi, yin and yang, and more) and exotic names for various positions (Opening Qi Door, Swan Stretches Her Wings, and others), qigong's ancient tried-and-true techniques can sometimes be hard for Westerners to grasp. In this book, I demystify and clarify the essence of qigong, providing you with useful tips to help you get the most out of your practice.

My studies of qigong began thirty years ago in San Francisco. I have been fortunate to learn from wonderful teachers, all of them men. As a female practitioner, I have taken the best of what qigong masters offered and modified some of what I learned to suit my needs. When I began teaching qigong myself, I developed these variations for the special needs and different energies of the women I taught. My approach in this book has been to take the best of the ancient tradition and synthesize it for the modern, Western woman. Each set in this book is based on centuries-old movements and the majority are presented exactly as I was taught them. Most of the exercises retain their traditional names, but I have given certain exercises new names to evoke the qualities I felt they nurture. Most importantly, I have carefully fine-tuned a sequence that fosters the vital energy of women. In short, I have brought my own personality and intuition to designing the workout and I hope you will do the same as you make this qigong practice your own.

The book is divided into three parts. Part One takes you posture by posture through the simple, graceful, energizing Twenty-Minute Workout. Postures are grouped into sets that take from thirty seconds to four minutes each, and there are seven sets in all. When you first begin your practice, Part One is all you really need to begin reaping the benefits of qigong.

Part Two helps you fine-tune your practice and deepen your understanding by explaining the benefits of each set of movements in greater detail. Here you will learn more about the philosophy behind qigong and how correct practice of the postures helps prevent illness, stops the progression of disease, strengthens and detoxifies vital organs, fortifies bones, stimulates lymphatic drainage, relieves stress, and promotes tranquility and vibrancy.

Part Three includes twenty-five categories of symptoms women commonly experience as they get older, identifying exercises from the Twenty-Minute Workout to help alleviate those symptoms. This section also goes beyond the core workout, presenting additional qigong postures and breathing techniques, self-acupressure, dietary suggestions, and self-massage techniques for alleviating specific concerns of mature women. This includes everything from maintaining bright eyes, soft skin, and healthy hair to building strong bones, reducing hot flashes, and improving sexual vitality.

True beauty comes from within and is manifested in that glow that accompanies a healthy body, mind, and spirit. For some women looking younger is important, but for others it doesn't much matter. Our common desire is to look and feel good. As Elizabeth Arden said, "I'm not interested in age. People who tell me their age are silly. You're as old as you feel." Indeed, it's not necessarily that we want to *be* young, just that we want to *feel* young.

As you practice qigong, you will be learning to "work your qi" to achieve this goal. Be aware that a qi workout requires concentration, and don't worry about what you look like as you exercise. People who know me as someone with a gentle expression who is often smiling tell me that I look so serious when I practice qigong. That's because taking care of oneself is serious business! The energy you cultivate during your practice will soon carry over into your everyday life and others are sure to notice the change in your appearance. More important, you will *feel* the difference.

No matter what your health and fitness goals, qigong can help you achieve them in a balanced, gentle way. The exercises and techniques presented in this book may be new for you, but they take very little time, are low impact, and easy to learn. What's more, you can do them in the privacy of your own home. It is my hope that when you embrace my simple workout plan, you will begin to experience the joys of looking and feeling your personal best, becoming, with every minute you practice qigong, truly ageless.

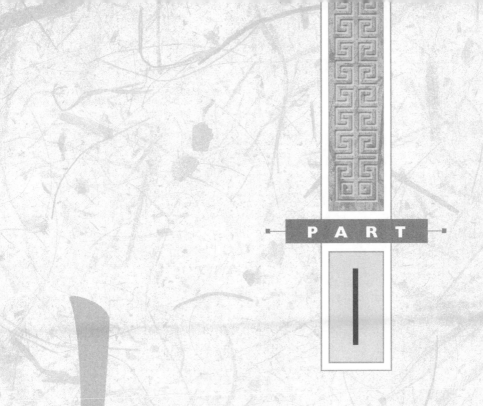

Living the Twenty-Minute Workout

Teachers open the door,
but you must enter by yourself.

CHINESE PROVERB

Use the mind to direct the qi.
Use the qi to propel the body.

CHANG SAN FENG,

TAI CHI CH'UAN CLASSICS

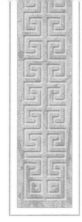

Starting Your Qigong Workout

THE FOLLOWING answers to common questions I get from my students will help you begin your qigong practice on the right foot.

How often do I need to practice qigong?

Qigong is most beneficial when you practice on a regular basis. Practicing every day is ideal, but it is fine to practice three times or even once a week. Whatever you are able to do, feel good about your choice. You may find that the more you practice, the more you want to practice. Qigong is enjoyable and doesn't require a huge amount of time, special equipment, or a large workout space. Practice your whole life for good health and longevity. Many people in China practice every day into their nineties and even past a hundred.

What type of environment do I need for my qigong practice?

The room temperature should be moderate, not too hot or too cold, with good ventilation and no strong fragrances or odors. Make sure you're not exercising where there is a draft. Choose a suitable time of day and a quiet room or a tranquil area outdoors. Practice outdoors in the fresh air whenever possible. This way, you will gather qi from nature.

What type of clothing should I wear?

Wear loose, comfortable cotton clothing without any restrictions, especially around the waist. Wear comfortable, flexible shoes. You can wear light sneakers or Chinese-style slippers, or even bare feet as long as your feet are warm.

What are the do's and don'ts of qigong practice?

Aim to maintain a consistent, regular practice.

Tradition dictates that you practice at sunrise, midday, or sunset. But anytime that works for you will do.

Don't eat or drink anything (especially cold drinks) within fifteen minutes before or after your qigong sessions.

Avoid talking while you practice.

Perform exercises in the order presented.

Don't overdo your practice. Too much of anything can be counterproductive.

Do the exercises based on your own abilities and health status.

If you get sore from any of the exercises, cut back. If soreness continues, consult your physician.

Don't rush through your practice.

Approach your practice with a positive attitude.

Bring your own style and personality to the practice.

Be patient with yourself. Realize it takes time to master the movements.

As you learn, you may choose to concentrate on one set of exercises per week, extending the length of time you practice.

You may vary the tempo of your practice each day. Some days you will want to move faster and other days more slowly.

Don't be concerned about finishing all of the sets in one workout if you are moving particularly slowly on a given day.

It is absolutely acceptable to take twenty minutes to do even one or two of these exercises.

Breathe naturally unless otherwise instructed.

MOVING BREATH

The coordination of the movement with your breathing gives you the first hint of what qigong exercise is all about. Moving with your breath creates a connection with the yang and yin forces of heaven and earth. "Heaven" refers to the Chinese concept of the yang healing power of the stars, moon, sun, and other heavenly aspects of our natural universe. "Earth" refers to the yin healing power of rivers, oceans, lakes, trees, rocks, soil, and mountains. When you coordinate breath and movement, you begin to feel your body as an integrated whole, deeply connected to all of nature.

To quiet your thoughts, count your breaths. Count an inhalation and exhalation as one breath. You will take approximately five deep breaths per minute. This is the ideal, and you may find yourself taking considerably more breaths per minute as a beginner. As you become more proficient, it won't be necessary to count breaths to clear the mind.

The speed and duration of your breath varies depending upon the type of movement you are doing. This explains the variations in number of breaths taken and time it takes to do a particular exercise. The suggested times and number of breaths I provide for each exercise are approximations and merely serve as a guide. Remember that the real guide comes from within—so make sure to listen carefully to yourself.

If you have difficulty with the breathing instructions due to limitations of your breathing capacity, you may want to try the following: take two complete deep breaths with the movement whenever the directions call for one complete deep breath. With time, your breathing capacity will most likely improve and you can then follow the regular instructions. (See page 177, *Breathing into Beautiful Belly*.)

We all have a tendency to rush our movements. To slow down, you might find it helpful to count in your mind as you breathe. A good rule of thumb is to count up to six on an inhalation and six on an exhalation.

As mentioned, slow, deep breaths add up to approximately five complete breaths per minute. This means that one breath takes about twelve seconds and you will have taken approximately 100 breaths by the time you finish the workout. Numbers aside, the most important thing is that you breathe deeply and comfortably, and that your movements are slow and gentle.

Allow the energy within to flow and your qigong practice will renew your body, mind, and spirit.

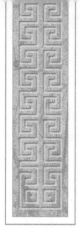

Warm-Up: Waking Up Qi

6

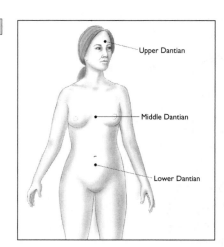

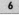 *Three Dantians*

THESE warm-up exercises promote the smooth circulation of qi, slowing degeneration and maintaining health, especially of your joints, muscles, and tendons. They also stimulate the flow of qi in the lower *dantian* (pronounced "don-tee-en"), an important reservoir of qi located below your navel and a key center of physical healing in the body. The lower *dantian* is often referred to as simply the *dantian*. There are, however, a total of three energy reservoirs: the lower, middle, and upper *dantian*. Each will be described more fully in the course of the workout.

As you do the warm-up, breathe naturally into your lower *dantian*. To breathe into the *dantian*, concentrate your mind on the area two inches below your belly button and into your abdomen toward your lower back. Breathing naturally, your belly expands upon inhalation and contracts during exhalation. As you learn to concentrate on your *dantian*, your energy drops to the lower part of your body. If you have ever been pregnant, you may recognize this as similar to the sensation of energy gathering in this area. Your *dantian* is a place of life and healing. The more you can concentrate on it, the more relaxed you will feel. Your shoulders relax, your breath capacity increases, and you feel a tremendous sense of grounding and centering within yourself. Concentrating your mind's attention on your *dantian,* you may also feel a heaviness and tingling in this area, which signifies that qi is circulating.

❁ Beautiful Woman Turns at Waist *(20 seconds)*

Stand with your feet together. Place your palms on the small of your back with fingers pointing downward. Begin making gentle clockwise circles with your waist. As you do the movement, visualize yourself standing in the center of a barrel. Your hips are moving around the circumference of the barrel. Be careful not to bend your knees with each rotation, but don't lock them either. They will naturally flex a little, but the movement stems from your waist, not from your shoulders or knees. Relax and flow with the circling movement of your hips. You will feel the energy beginning to stir in your *dantian.*

As you feel the bottoms of your feet being massaged, know that you are stimulating the health of your internal organs. Let this gentle circular movement remind you of the importance of connecting with yourself and the earth beneath you. This movement also teaches you how important it is to protect and nourish your lower back and gives you a sensation of gently

● *Beautiful Woman Turns at Waist*

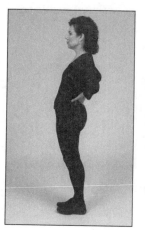
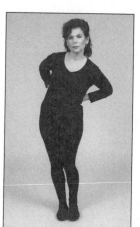
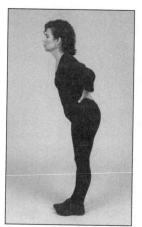
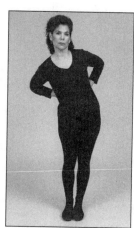

building, never-ending energy so pleasant you may feel as if you never want to stop!

Make six full clockwise circles and then six full counterclockwise circles.

❀ Beautiful Woman Turns at Hips *(20 seconds)*

Stand with your feet shoulder-width apart and parallel, tailbone tucked under and belly soft. Rest your palms with fingers facing downward on your hip sockets. Make wide circles with your hips.

Beautiful Woman Turns at the Hips give you a sensation that your lower body is swinging freely as your hips open and become increasingly flexible. As you form large circles, any qi stagnation in the hip and ankle joints is released. With this movement, you become even more aware of your belly. As you circle, relax your shoulders and let your energy continue to drop into the belly.

Concentrate on your *dantian* and allow all movement to evolve from the hips, not knees or shoulders. Make sure that your legs are fairly wide apart so you can make big circles.

Remember that your mind guides your qi and where you mind goes, your qi follows. In qigong, many of our movements stem from the *dantian,* which is like the middle of a wheel, the energy hub around which all movements circulate. Concentrating on and moving from the *dantian* creates a fluidity throughout the body and a connection of each part of your body to the whole.

Practice six times clockwise and six times counterclockwise.

● *Beautiful Woman Turns at Hips*

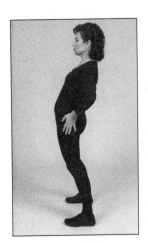
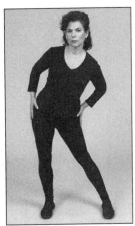
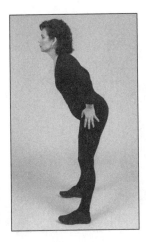
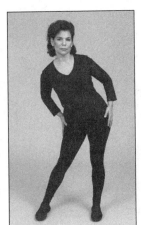

❈ Circling Knees *(15 seconds)*

Stand with your feet together flat on the floor, and your legs touching. Bend your knees at approximately a forty-five-degree angle, or as close to that as you comfortably can, resting your palms on your bent knees. Keep your back straight. Begin making small circles parallel to the ground with your knees level.

Because you are exerting yourself a bit more here than you have in the two previous exercises, you may find yourself holding your breath. Breathe naturally and concentrate on making whole, level circles. Relax your shoulders. Feel the flexibility in your ankle joints and the strong sensation that gravity is pulling you toward the earth. As you move, keep your knees at the same height. Refrain from bobbing up and down or you will strain your knees. Keep your buttocks low, your head raised and your gaze steady. Move mainly your knees, letting the rest of your body follow naturally.

If you have knee problems, be cautious doing this exercise. Gently rest your hands on your knees to support your knee joints. Do fewer repetitions when you first begin practicing. Add more circles as your quadriceps and hamstring muscles become stronger. If this exercise is a challenge for you at first, you will find that with practice it becomes easier and more enjoyable.

Practice six times clockwise and six times counterclockwise.

● *Circling Knees*

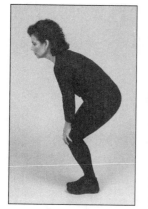 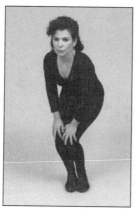 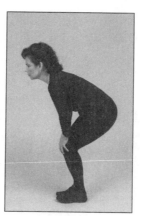 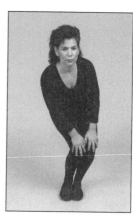

NOTE ‖ Some of my students move their knees out in opposite directions when they do Circling Knees, resembling flappers from the Roaring Twenties. I encourage you to practice both ways, legs moving together and in opposite directions. Each works the muscles of the legs in a different way.

❀ Monkey Stretches Up and Down *(30 seconds)*

Stand with your knees straight but not locked and your feet together. Interlace your fingers with your palms cupped upward in front of your waist. Inhale and raise your clasped hands, keeping your wrists straight. As your hands come level with your chest, turn your palms outward. Raise your arms above your head and turn your face to the sky. Continue pushing upward toward the sky as you complete your inhalation. Exhale, still clasping the hands, and ro-

● *Monkey Stretches Up and Down*

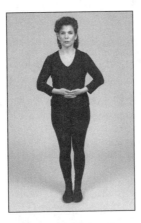
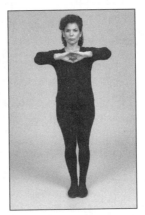
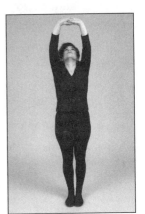
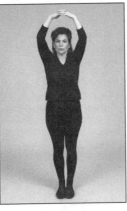
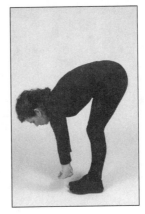
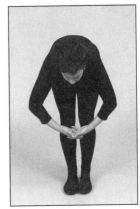

tate your palms downward. Lower your arms along the same path in front of your body and bend at the waist. Bend your elbows so your arms are close to your body as you lower toward the ground. Bending over, maintain a flat back, and stretch both arms toward your toes. With your palms and gaze facing the earth, complete your exhalation.

Inhaling, turn your clasped hands inward and then upward, retracing the movement back toward the sky. This exercise creates a wonderful stretch in your back, opening the spaces between each vertebra and creating a feeling of great openness. Not only are you stretching your back but you are releasing blockages throughout your *entire* body—stimulating nearly every single joint, your arms, torso, and the backs of your legs. As you stretch up and down, tension is released within your shoulder joints and you may notice qi flowing into your hands. As you stretch up to the heavens and down to the earth, feel the qi emanating from a point at the center of each palm known as *laogong* (see illustration on page 20). The *laogong* point is a special center of energy transmission in qigong.

Practice up and down three times, a total of three complete breaths.

Helpful Hint

If you have trouble touching the ground when stretching downward, just hang over as far as you can go. As you hang, concentrate on loosening your tight muscles. Take three deep breaths as you visualize the tight muscle relaxing, stretching, and releasing. When ready, rise slowly, rolling upward one vertebra at a time until you return to a standing position. Gradually, you will notice your stretch deepen.

If you are suffering from lower back pain or injury, stretch extra slowly and gently. Don't go any farther than feels absolutely comfortable and be sure to ask the advice of your health-care professional.

✿ Opening Qi Door *(5 seconds)*

This exercise and the following two are a triad. All three target free flow of energy within the shoulders, arms, wrists, and hands. For all three, stand in Horse Stance, feet parallel and wider than your shoulders, hands on waist,

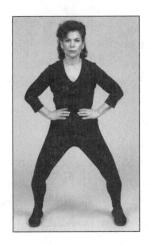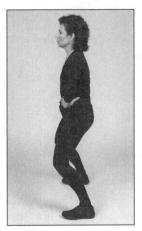

● *Horse Stance*

head erect, buttocks tucked under, and back straight. Your knees are bent out over your feet and remain so for the duration of the exercises.

To open the qi door, stretch your arms straight out in front of you at shoulder level. With your palms facing upward, bend your elbows and draw your arms back underneath your armpits. Your elbows are behind your body, your bent arms close to your sides and your fingertips close together and stretching forward.

Extend your hands out in front of you as you straighten your arms again. Turn your palms to face each other, about six inches apart. Stretch your fingertips upward toward the sky and then flex and extend your wrists as far as you comfortably can, holding your thumbs and fingers close together but not touching.

Begin opening your imaginary qi door with the fingers of both hands. Your fingers spread apart one by one in a fanlike motion in front of you. The fingers of your right hand move clockwise, the fingers of your left hand, counterclockwise.

Once your fingers circle around to the bottom and the qi door is open, bring your hands in toward your body with palms open and up. Imagine you are holding a ball of qi as your hands draw back in toward your body. Bend your elbows and bring your bent arms once again to each side of your body. With your hands open and palms facing upward, draw your hands underneath your armpits again.

With this movement, you draw qi in to your middle *dantian*, the energy reserve located in your chest. As the energy of the universal life force floods

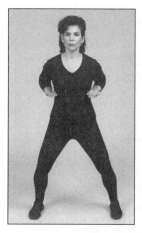
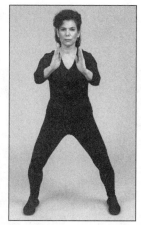
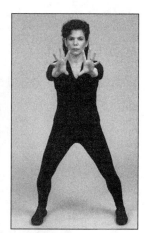

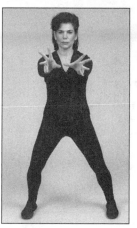
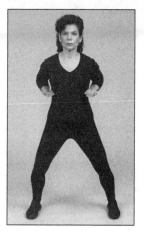

● *Opening Qi Door*

into your middle *dantian,* feel it spread up, down, and throughout your whole body like a sunburst.

Practice three times.

❋ Flapping Wrists *(3 seconds)*

Remaining in Horse Stance, extend your hands out in front of you at shoulder height, palms and fingertips facing and six inches apart. This is an isolated movement of your hands and wrists. Your arms do not move. They are stationary and steady, with a slight bend in your elbows. Allow your hands to flap quickly as if they are fast-moving flippers in a pinball machine. Repeat the same motion with your palms facing downward. The wrists are totally relaxed

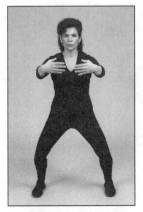
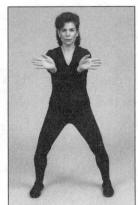

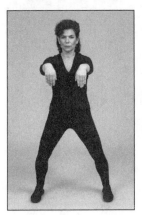
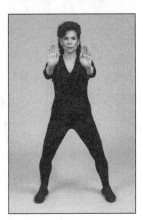

● *Flapping Wrists*

while the hands flap in and out, and then up and down. To protect your wrist joints, be careful not to flap too vigorously.

This movement can bring a smile to your face, maybe because it tickles your funny bone. As you flap, any constraint in the joints of your hands falls away. The shoulders, though they do not move, are also stimulated, as is your brain. Notice the vibration through the wrists, up the arm and into the shoulders to your brain. This vibration releases toxins and toxic emotions from your body, cleansing you on all levels.

Flap back and forth nine times in each position.

❀ Separating Clouds *(5 seconds)*

Remain in Horse Stance and lower your arms. Cross your hands at the wrists, palms facing your *dantian.* In this movement, you will trace the circumference

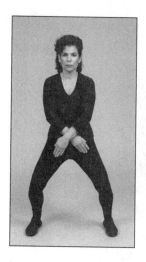 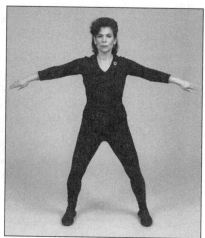 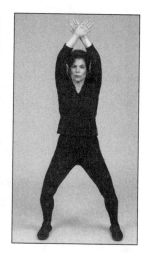

of a large circle in one fast, continuous motion. Begin at your *dantian*, then separate your hands and bring them down to your sides. Swing your arms out wide behind you and up in a circle toward the sky until they meet and cross above your head. Continuing to trace the circle in front of you, lower your arms and end with your hands crossed at your *dantian*. As your arms move out and away from your body, your chest opens and you feel your rib cage expand, providing a tremendous release of the tightness you hold here. As your arms circle inward, your chest contracts. Make wide, rapid circles to increase circulation in your shoulder joints. Then reverse the direction of your arms.

● *Separating Clouds*

This movement can be quite a challenge for the brain when it comes to switching directions. Just let your arms fly without thinking about it and you will be rewarded with a wonderful release from the tension held in the shoulders.

Practice each direction three times.

❋ Brushing Wind *(7 seconds)*

Stand comfortably with your feet about a foot apart and knees slightly bent. Rest your hands comfortably at your sides. Think of yourself as a marionette doll with strings attached to your wrists. Raise your arms quickly upward, leading with the topsides of your wrists as if they were being pulled up by the strings. Keep your hands limp with fingertips pointing downward and your arms slightly bent. End this movement with your arms at shoulder height.

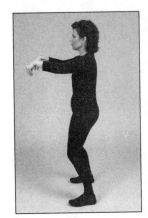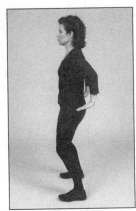

● *Brushing Wind*

Now reverse the movement, letting your arms relax and drop downward. Keep your arms relatively straight with just a slight bend at the elbows. Your wrists are flexed and the heels of your hands lead, fingertips following behind, elbows pointing down and shoulders relaxed. Swing arms downward until your hands are a few inches behind your sides. At this point, both elbows are partially bent and palms push straight toward the ground.

Opening Qi Door brought qi into your body and Flapping Wrists and Separating Clouds got qi moving throughout your body. With Brushing Wind, you are grounded and relaxed. There is a sensation that your whole body is connected from the top of your head down to bottoms of your feet, a great flow of qi all along this axis. As you do this movement, notice how strong your torso feels. With this simple movement, you present yourself to the world as strong and capable, your movement springing from a boundless supply of qi.

Do the upward and downward motion six times.

NOTE ‖ Make sure your hands don't go above shoulder height, which would create too much tension in your shoulder joints and limit the amount of qi flowing into your hands.

❁ Phoenix Eats Its Ashes *(10 seconds)*

Now that you feel capable of anything, you are ready for a real challenge! Stand with your weight on your left leg and your right heel resting on the ground in front of you. Your left foot turns outward at a forty-five degree angle. Your right ankle is flexed with your toes pointing to the sky. Bend your left knee out over your left foot, and extend your right leg out in front of you, your heel sliding along the ground. Bend at your waist and stretch over your right leg. Grasp your upturned foot and pull it toward your chin without lifting your right heel from the ground. Stretch your neck and attempt to bring your chin to your toes. Keep your back straight and extend your buttocks way back as you stretch the hamstring of your right thigh. Lengthen your back by stretching your torso straight out from hip. Breathe naturally! You will feel an incredible stretch on the back of your leg. Maintain a flat back. Practicing this exercise at night when your muscles are least tight can improve your flexibility. It is definitely a "stretch" to accomplish this movement with good form. But the benefits far outweigh the extra effort required. This is commitment! Remember to breathe.

Repeat on your left side. Practice once on each side.

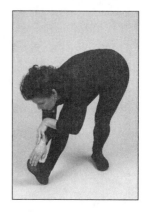

● *Phoenix Eats Its Ashes*

NOTE ‖ As impossible as it sounds, the goal of this exercise is to actually touch your chin to your toes. But don't worry if you don't quite make it, and don't strain too much. Great benefits can be experienced either way.

❀ Tigress Crouches Down *(5 seconds)*

Begin by standing with both feet flat on the ground, parallel to each other and wider than shoulder-width apart. Bend your left knee as deeply as you can and stretch your right leg out to the side. Rest your hands on your thighs. The ideal is to keep a straight back and stay as upright as possible, although it is natural to lean forward a bit to keep your balance. As much as possible, maintain a straight back and a straight outstretched leg. In this position, notice gravity pulling you down to the earth from the perineum point (midway between your vagina and anus, see illustration page 174). You may notice energy shooting up through this point all the way to the Hundred Meeting point at the top of your head (see illustration on page 88). The more you can relax into this stretch, the more revived and revitalized you will feel.

Practice once on each side.

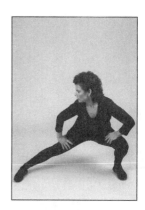

● *Tigress Crouches Down*

If you are having trouble maintaining your balance or need a better stretch in this position, hold on to a piece of furniture, a fence, a bench, a bar or anything else low enough to help you sink into the position with a straight back. Stand in front of your support and as close to it as possible. Start with your feet together, holding on to your support. Slowly bend both knees as deeply as you can, keeping your feet close together and flat on the floor. Shift your weight backward a little. Then extend your right leg out to the side, holding on to the support. Stretch and hold that position for a few minutes. Relax into your hip and work to get your extended foot flat on the ground as you gently stretch your ankle joint. Only when you are ready, bring your right leg in so it is once again bent next to your left leg. Switch sides. This helps to gradually open up the hip and ankle joints and strengthens the muscles of your lower back.

When doing this exercise it's not a matter of how low can you go. The key is to maintain proper posture to ensure the smooth flow of qi within your muscles, tendons, joints, and ligaments. Don't force the movement. Instead, imagine your qi sinking downward as your torso lowers toward the earth. Release all of the tension in your body as you do this and soon you will find yourself almost "falling" downward (this posture is also referred to as the Falling Stance, but that doesn't mean your goal is to literally fall to the floor!).

Warning: Doing this exercise as described above can prevent injuries to the knees. But if you have knee problems, take extra care to avoid going too low. Placing your hands on top of your knees as you bend them provides extra support. Always know your own limitations and absolutely listen to your body as you move through your qigong practice.

❋ Concluding the Warm-Up *(15 seconds)*

Take time to notice any new sensations in your body. Stand or sit comfortably. Keep your spine straight, the crown of your head reaching upward, your tongue resting gently on the roof of your mouth. Let your mind be still. Notice your surroundings, watch your natural breathing, and take an "inventory" of your body, noticing any sensations. Begin the next exercise only when you are absolutely ready. Give yourself all the time you need. You deserve it. Although doing so will extend your workout slightly beyond twenty minutes, consider taking some time between all the sets to "check in" with yourself in this way.

This completes the warm-up. Your qi is now awake!

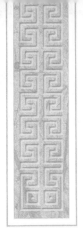

Set I: Tapping for Qi

20

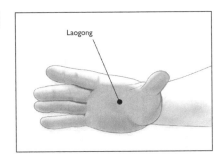

Laogong

● Laogong Point

THIS brief set stimulates and nourishes the qi of your internal organs, lymphatic system, energy pathways, and brain with a revitalizing self-massage in the form of tapping. The more attention we give to these structures, the healthier we are. When you tap, you stimulate the flow of qi by stimulating acupressure points along your body. As you gently and gradually increase the force and speed of your hands, you feel the qi build up throughout your system. As you begin the tapping described in each exercise, bring your attention to the particular area and organ system you are stimulating. Qi follows your attention, so directing your mind in this way helps enhance qi flow, dissolving blocks.

In addition to varying the speed with which you tap, you may also choose to experiment with different hand positions. Tap with an open hand, using your fingers, palm, back or side of the hand, or with a loose fist. Each hand position creates a different sensation. For example, tapping with an open palm is excellent for directing the qi that flows from your *dantian* through the important *laogong* acupressure point. Energy is believed to come in from the universe through this point and a person can also send qi from their body out through *laogong*.

No matter what hand position you choose, experiment and have fun feeling the qi coming into and going out from *laogong* and the pleasurable massage you are giving yourself as you tap.

❀ Rag Doll Twist *(7 seconds)*

Stand with your feet parallel and slightly wider than shoulder-width apart. Open your arms out to your sides at a forty-five-degree angle. Swing both of your arms to the right, your left arm crossing in front of your body and your right arm crossing behind your back. Allow your upper body to twist as it follows the motion of the arms. As you twist to the right, pivot your left foot inward on the toe. As your arms gently whip around, your left hand taps the right side of your torso, stimulating your liver and gallbladder; the back of your right hand taps the left side of your back, stimulating the left kidney.

Next, swing your arms to the left, allowing your upper body to twist as it follows the motion of the arms. As you twist to the left, your right foot pivots inward on the ball of your foot. As your arms whip gently around, your left hand hits your lower back on the right side, stimulating your right kidney; the palm of your right hand hits the area to the middle left of your torso, stimulating your stomach, spleen, and pancreas.

● *Rag Doll Twist*

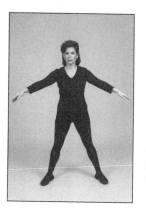 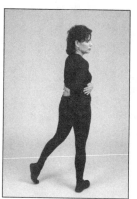 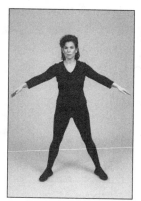 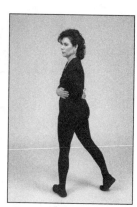

As you do this exercise, notice the heaviness and solid structure of your organs. Looking to the left and then the right, become aware, too, that you are balancing two sides of yourself. Notice the hardness of the movement when your hands hit your torso, and the softness as you twist from side to side. Swinging and tapping makes us aware of our torso, stimulating deeply the vital organs which carry out all our life functions and perking up our energy in the process.

Practice three times on each side.

❋ Thump Pump *(15 seconds)*

This exercise and the next one stimulate qi flow through your arms and legs. Stand with feet shoulder-width apart and parallel. Making a loose fist with your right hand, use the palm side of your hand to vigorously thump your left arm from the outside of your wrist up to the top of your shoulder. The motion is fast and relatively hard. You can even hear the thump sound made by the contact of your hand and body. Next, proceed down the inside of your arm from just below your armpit to the wrist. Change sides and repeat.

Become aware of any "congestion" you feel in your arms and legs. Some spots may be a little sore, and you can concentrate your massage in those areas. When you tap, feel the vibrations emanating throughout your whole body.

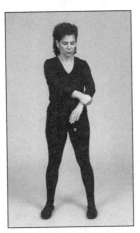 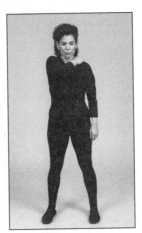 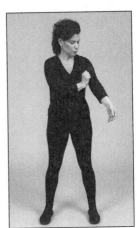

● *Outside of the Arm*　　● *Top of the Shoulders*　　● *Inside of the Arm*

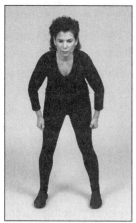
● *Outside of the Thighs*

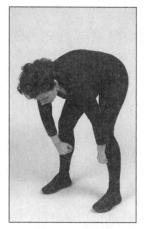
● *Inside of the Legs*

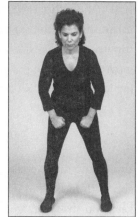
● *Inside of the Thighs*

Now use both hands simultaneously on your legs. Move first down the outsides of both legs to the feet and then up the inside to the upper thighs.

Next, thump the pressure points of your lymphatic system, which helps maintain a strong immune system by bringing nourishment to your cells and removing waste. Bend your knees slightly and gently thump the backs of both knees simultaneously. Next, stand up straight again and thump the area on your hip bone just above the creases in your legs, known as the inguinal groove. Use the opposite hand for each leg. Also, thump under each armpit and then on the side of your neck with the opposing hand. Change sides and repeat.

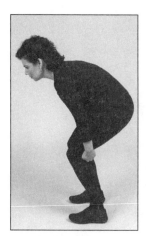
● *Backs of the Knees*

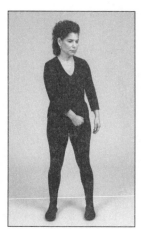
● *Inguinal Groove*

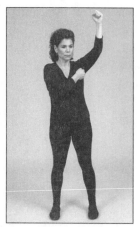
● *Under the Armpit*

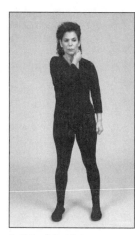
● *Side of the Neck*

Do this entire exercise once.

You will become more and more aware of your energy pathways being stimulated, the tension in your muscles being released, and your lymph being moved. Thumping is a great "waker-upper" when done by itself in the morning when you first get out of bed, releasing any kinks.

✿ Beating the Heavenly Drum *(8 seconds)*

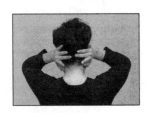

● *Beating Heavenly Drum*

You can do this exercise either standing or sitting. If standing, do so comfortably with feet about a foot apart, legs straight, knees slightly bent. If sitting, keep your back straight, legs uncrossed, and feet resting comfortably on the floor. To tune out noises, cover your ears with your palms. Lay your fingers flat on the base of your skull with your fingertips nearly meeting at the center. Use your ring, middle, and index fingers to quickly tap the back of your head where your skull meets your neck muscles. This area houses several important acupressure points. Quickly alternating between your three tapping fingers creates a sound just like a drum roll and promotes sharpness of the mind.

Not only will your mental processes get sharper as you tap but you will also feel your spine stimulated all the way down to your perineum.

Continue tapping until you have completed one full inhalation and exhalation. When you are finished, remove your hands from your ears slowly. Awaken, renewed, to your surroundings.

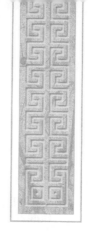

Set 2: Five Healing Sounds

THIS set promotes purification and nourishment of the internal organs through vocalization of five healing sounds. Each sound is related to one of the five major organs and the negative emotions associated with each:

- liver: anger
- heart: sadness
- spleen: worry
- lungs: grief
- kidneys: fear

When you make the sounds let them be soft and relaxed. Loud sounds cause tension in the organ, blocking qi circulation. After an inhalation, pause for a second and then release the organ sound in a continuous manner for the duration of your exhalation. As you inhale, bring good positive healing energy into the organ. As you exhale, visualize the release of the negative emotion.

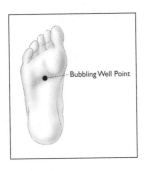

● *Bubbling Well Point*

Keep your eyes open during this exercise. Although the following description is for standing poses, the sounds can also be practiced sitting or lying down.

Helpful Hint

During these exercises, focus on the middle *dantian*. Allow the fresh, vital, clean qi to flow up the energy pathways in your legs via the toes or the Bubbling Well point at the bottoms of your feet. Feel energy travel up your legs, into your torso and chest, where it floods into the middle *dantian*.

It's not unusual for saliva to be created in the mouth during this set. Swallow the saliva slowly and visualize it passing down to your lower *dantian*. This is a precious bodily substance called "divine water" that can be used as internal medicine.

❀ *Shu—Liver* (20 seconds)

Stand comfortably, feet shoulder-width apart. Form fists with your hands and cross them at the wrists in front of your *dantian*. Begin your inhalation, moving your arms up in front of your body, keeping wrists crossed until they are above your head. Then separate your wrists, bringing your arms down and out to your sides as if tracing a large circle, keeping your hands still in fists. At the bottom of the circle, bring your forearms close together in front of your body with your hands facing upward and still in fists. Rest your elbows in front of your rib cage as you complete your inhalation.

● *Liver Healing Sound*

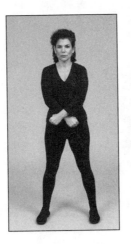
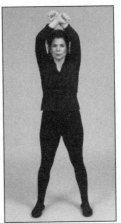
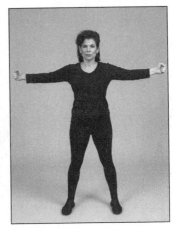

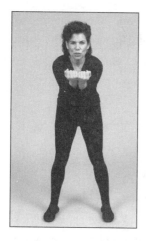
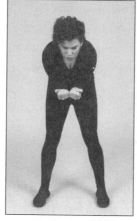

● *Liver Healing Sound*
(continued)

Begin your exhalation, releasing the sound *"shuuuu"* as you bend over slightly, keeping forearms together and elbows pressed lightly under your rib cage. This exercise releases the emotion of anger.

Practice three times for a total of three complete breaths.

✿ *Huhr—Heart* (30 seconds)

Stand comfortably with your feet shoulder-width apart, hands at your sides. Take a deep breath and bend your knees and elbows, forming fists and drawing your elbows in to your sides. As you exhale, you will raise your hands up and out into a wide V above you. Raise your hands over your head

● *Heart Healing Sound*

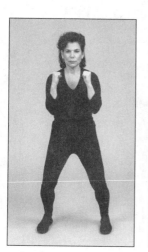
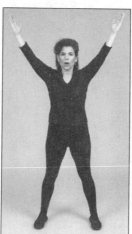

with your elbows pointing outward, your arms slightly rounded. As you raise your hands, open your fists gradually and exhale, emitting the sound *"huhrrrr."* End with your hands unfurled above your head, chest open. This exercise releases built-up toxins around your heart as well as the emotion of sadness.

Practice three times for a total of three complete breaths.

✿ *Hoo—Spleen* (20 seconds)

Stand comfortably with your feet together. With your palms facing downward, place the index finger of each hand at the front of your hips. Your fingertips are pointing to the center of your body. Keeping your elbows bent and your wrists flexed, take a deep breath and stretch your right hand upward and away from your body with palm pushing up toward the sky and fingertips pointing inward. Your left hand remains at your hip, pushing down toward the earth.

As you exhale, keep your hands and arms in the same position and twist your waist to the left. After twisting as far as you can, take a deep inhalation and hold it for ten seconds. Make the *"hooooo"* sound as you exhale, returning back toward center, while moving your right arm down diagonally across the front of your body. As you move your arm, rotate your wrist so that your palm turns toward you. When your hand reaches hip level, draw your right

● *Spleen Healing Sound*

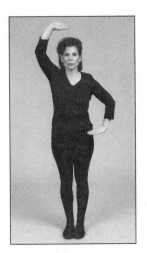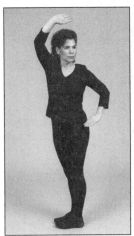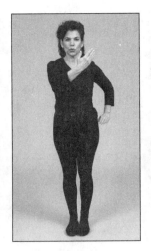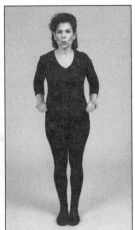

elbow, palm up, back into your body until your pinky touches the side of your hip. Turn your left hand upward so that it is in the same position as your right hand. This exercise releases toxins from your spleen and eliminates worry from your mind.

Practice one time, on one side only, for a total of two complete breaths.

✿ See-*ah*—Lungs *(20 seconds)*

Stand with your feet slightly wider than shoulder-width apart and either parallel or open at a forty-five-degree angle. Inhale and bend slightly at the waist, reaching your hands downward as if you are scooping qi up from the earth. Imagine that you are gathering a big fluffy pile of leaves. Your palms are facing each other, your arms are rounded, and you can feel the qi coming into your hands, arms, and *dantian.* Continuing your inhalation, pull your arms in toward your body, bending at the elbows with palms facing you until they reach shoulder level. Next, turn your palms outward at a slight angle, fingertips facing up and fingers close together. With the outer edge of your hands leading the movement, exhale and emit the sound *"see-ahhhh"* as you press your hands out in front of you at a forty-five-degree angle. Extend your arms as far as they can go and bend your knees slightly out over your feet. This exercise detoxifies and purifies your lungs and releases the emotion of grief.

Practice three times for a total of three complete breaths.

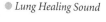 *Lung Healing Sound*

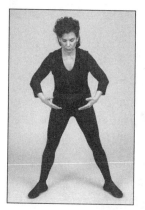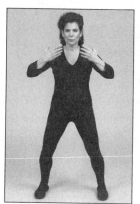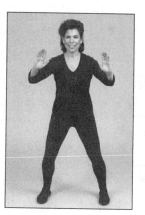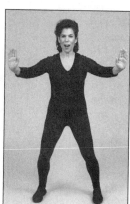

✿ Cherwee—Kidneys *(30 seconds)*

Stand comfortably with your feet shoulder-width apart. Rest the backs of both hands on your lower back, making a loose fist with each hand. Rub your lower back in small circles where your kidneys reside. Breathe naturally.

Then, on your inhalation, draw your hands up both sides of your body until your hands are at your armpits. Relax your fists, but keep your fingertips curled inward. On your exhalation, release the sound *"cherweeee"* gently and softly from your vocal cords as you extend your arms in front of you with your hands facing your chest, palms facing in toward your heart, fingertips about six inches apart. This detoxifies your kidneys and releases the emotion of fear.

Practice three times for a total of three complete breaths.

● *Kidney Healing Sound*

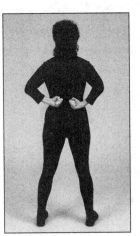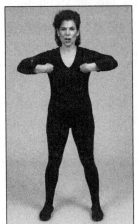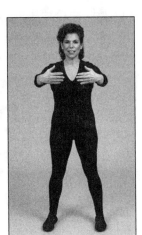

✿ Five Healing Sounds Finale *(15 seconds)*

End this group of exercises by gathering and storing the energy you have generated in your middle *dantian.* Relax your arms at your sides and allow any sensations to surface as you concentrate on the five organs you've stimulated. Send love and appreciation to all of these organs. Next, place the palms of both hands over your middle *dantian,* your right hand covered by your left. Stand for a few moments and send the energy from your hands into your middle *dantian.* Feel the sense of peace flow throughout your entire being as you connect with your qi and your heart. Do for one or two deep breaths.

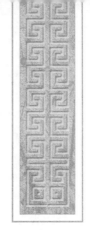

Set 3: Playing with Qi

4 MINUTES

THE THIRD set contains basic movements designed to acquaint you with your qi as it flows through the various meridians, or energy pathways, in your body. The simple movements are coordinated with your slow, gentle breath and allow you to feel the warmth and texture of your qi as it ebbs and flows from one movement to the next. All of the movements in this set are performed slowly, rhythmically, and gracefully. To get yourself to slow down, you might find it helpful to count in your mind as you breathe.

❋ Feeling Qi *(1 minute 30 seconds)*

During this exercise, stand with your feet shoulder-width apart and your knees slightly bent, arms at your sides. You may also choose to sit in a chair with your feet flat on the floor and your back straight.

To prepare, direct your gaze in a diagonal line to a point in front of you, about five feet down from the tip of your nose. This gaze is called the Taoist Plumb Line. Focusing your eyes in this way helps you to concentrate your attention inward and to connect with your internal qi flow. Your back is straight and your knees are slightly bent, your spine flat and relaxed in the lumbar region, and your fingers spread apart so qi can move from one hand into the other.

Bring your hands in front of your stomach and rub them together quickly, creating friction and heat between them. Then rub the center of each palm with the opposite thumb in a circular movement, bringing more vital energy into your hands through the *laogong* point. Do this for the length of one deep, complete breath.

Now it is time to begin Feeling Qi. Place your hands in front of your *dantian* with palms facing each other as if you are holding a small imaginary ball there. As you visualize this ball, you may begin to feel a heat or tingling between your hands. This is qi. Play with this energy by opening and closing your hands. Feel this imaginary qi ball expand and contract between your hands. Notice the different sensations that arise. You may experience a sense of heaviness, a pulling and pushing, tingling, heat, buoyancy, blowing air, electricity, or some other sensation that you can't even describe in words. These are all indications that qi is moving between your hands. If you don't feel anything, don't worry—the qi is still there!

Allow your hands to relax as they hold the expanding and contracting qi ball. Move your hands closer and farther away from each other as you wish, but do not let them touch each other. Move them higher and wider, but not higher than shoulder level. Breathe in as your hands move out or up and breathe out when your hands move in or down.

● *Feeling Qi*   Move hands in and out six times for a total of six complete breaths.

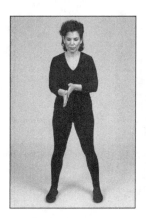 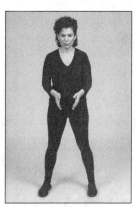 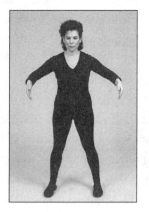 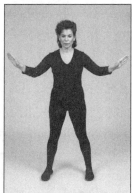

Helpful Hint

Make certain your wrists and shoulders are relaxed during this exercise. If your wrists (and/or shoulders) are tense during your practice your hands will remain cold or you may not experience any sensations between them. Do not cup your hands as if they could hold water. Instead, hold your palms loosely and slightly rounded as if water could flow out of them.

❋ Fluffing White Clouds *(1 minute 15 seconds)*

Stand with your feet parallel, shoulder-width apart with your knees slightly bent. Your hands are resting open at your sides with your pinky fingers next to your legs and fingertips facing the earth. As you inhale, straighten your knees and lift your hands to shoulder height in front of you with palms facing upward and elbows slightly bent.

As you exhale, turn your palms downward and bring your arms down, drawing your wrists back in toward your body and bending your knees again. The heel of your hand leads and fingertips follow. End with elbows slightly bent, palms face downward, your hands by your sides stretched out flat as if gently patting white clouds. Turn your palms upward and continue from the beginning. Coordinate the movement of your hands with the bending and straightening of your legs.

The sensation of qi during this exercise can be extraordinary. As your

● *Fluffing White Clouds*

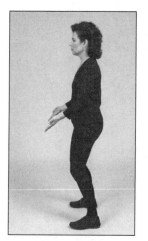
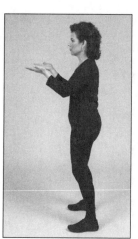
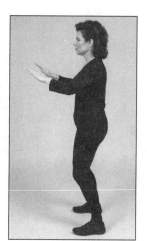
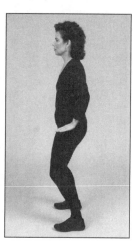

palms move upward, you may feel they hold a heavy weight. This is abundant qi from the universe. By contrast, when your palms turn down and float back to your sides, it may feel as if there is a light, fluffy pillow beneath them. The power of these sensations increases with every repetition of the movement and your deep, rhythmical breath.

Practice up and down six times for a total of six complete breaths.

✿ Swan Stretches Her Wings *(1 minute 15 seconds)*

With Feeling Qi, you experienced qi moving along the horizontal axis. Fluffing Clouds gave you a sense of qi's vertical motion. Swan Stretches Her Wings stimulates qi across both the horizontal and vertical axes of your body, connecting you to the earth and the heavens and unifying both your right and left sides. Stretching and opening, you feel that the universe is providing you with everything you need.

Stand comfortably with your feet together and your hands at your sides. With your palms facing downward, place the index finger of each hand at the front of your hips, your fingertips pointing to the center of your body. Keeping your elbow bent and your wrist flexed, inhale and stretch your right hand up and away from your body, palm pushing up toward the sky and fingertips pressed together and pointing in toward your head. Your left hand remains at your hip, simultaneously pushing down toward the earth. Your elbows are slightly bent and your shoulders relaxed as both arms curve across your body.

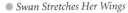
● *Swan Stretches Her Wings*

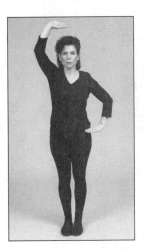
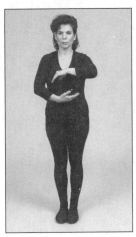
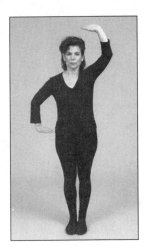

In one continuous motion, turn both palms to face each other then, as you exhale, lower your right arm along the same path you raised it. Gliding your right hand around the side of an imaginary qi ball resting between your middle and lower *dantians,* simultaneously raise your left arm and glide it around the other side of the ball. Bring your right hand around to cup the bottom of the ball and your left hand to the top. Next, as your hands break apart, inhale and raise your left hand to the sky as you push your right hand to the earth, reversing your stretch and the curve of your arms across your body. Now bring your arms down to form the ball with your hands again, this time with the left hand under and the right hand cradling the top of the ball. The hand facing the sky always comes underneath the ball.

Alternate three times on each side for a total of six complete breaths.

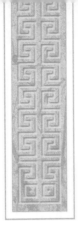

Set 4: Qi Mind, Qi Body

THE EXERCISES in this set focus the intent of our minds and open and strengthen our connection with the dynamic forces of nature that nourish and nurture us as women.

❋ Woman Connects with Heaven and Earth
(30 seconds)

Stand with your feet wider than shoulder-width apart and pointing out at a forty-five-degree angle. Keep your back straight, head erect, and buttocks tucked under. Concentrate on the bottoms of your feet and feel them connecting with the surface you are standing on. Imagine your soles reaching through and connecting to the earth as if they have roots growing into the ground. Imagine that you are soaking up water from the earth and it is nourishing your entire body. Inhale and touch the backs of your hands together, fingertips leading down. Gently squat, bending your knees until they extend out over your toes.

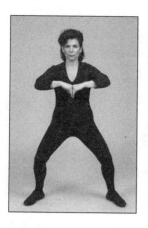 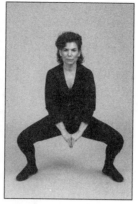

● Downward Movement

Move slowly and stay relaxed, maintaining a straight back. Make certain not to lean over. Continue lowering your body in this position as low as you comfortably can. As you bend, maintain the positions of your hands with the backs of the hands touching and fingertips pointing downward as if you are dipping them into a sea of qi. Straighten your arms, your fingers moving down the center of your body. Your inhalation ends when you reach your lowest point.

Begin your upward movement toward the heavens with a slow, gradual exhalation. Slowly straighten your knees and move your hands up, fingers still pointing downward. When your hands reach your middle *dantian,* separate them and gradually move them up and out until they stretch over your head. As you stretch your fingers toward the heavens, your palms face each other.

Feel your chest open as you raise your arms and notice the qi between the middle of your palms. As your hands reach up and over your head, arch your

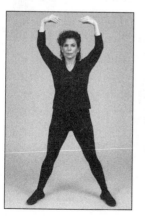 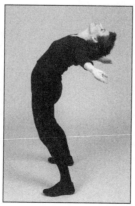

● Upward Movement

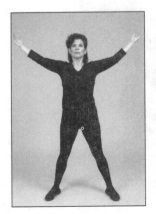
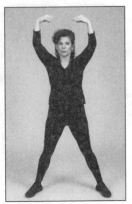
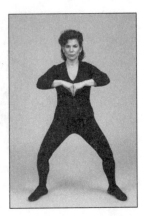

● *Retrace Downward Movement*

back and allow your arms to fall back open behind you. Surrender back as far as you comfortably can, maintaining your balance as you complete your exhalation.

Retrace the movement as you begin your inhalation and come out of the backward bend. Bring your hands toward each other above your head until they are touching back to back once again. Bend down as your hands move slowly along the center of your body, first past the middle and then to your lower *dantian*. This completes one cycle of the movement. Continue inhaling and repeat the movement from the beginning, exhaling again as you move upward.

Practice three times for a total of three complete breaths.

❀ Yi-Chuan Standing and Walking

Yi-Chuan is a qigong system of standing and walking exercises, and is known as the style of no style. It allows you to draw the force of the universe into yourself in order to foster your natural, instinctive abilities. This practice, described in the next two exercises, brings you in touch with the yin and yang energies that create balance within your mind, body, and spirit. Standing Like a Tree is a form of Yi-Chuan standing, while Walking Like a Turtle is a form of Yi-Chuan walking.

❇ Standing Like a Tree *(1 minute)*

The eight standing postures described below promote mental awareness, help you absorb healthy, abundant qi from the environment, and promote toxin release. They also help you to experience the expansion of your whole body upon inhalation and contraction of your body all at once upon exhalation.

All the Standing Like a Tree postures are done with your feet parallel and a bit wider than your shoulders, knees slightly bent. With a straight back and relaxed chin, look out into the distance. Experience the sensation of your entire body expanding and contracting with each breath. As you stand, you may notice energy flowing in your torso and palms. Feel the fullness in your fingertips. Concentrate on the *laogong* point as you root yourself to the ground. Relax all of your joints to allow qi to flow freely and with abundance.

Quiet your thoughts and concentrate on your breath.

On your inhalation, straighten your posture slightly and expand your chest as you allow your qi to expand outward and ascend. On your exhalation, relax your body and chest and allow your qi to descend. As you do this notice a sense of firmness in your *dantian* and allow the weight of your body to sink lower.

HELPFUL HINTS FOR ALIGNING YOUR CENTER

■ Bend your knees slightly so you can't see your feet. The deeper you bend your knees while keeping your back straight, the greater the benefits. Do not lock your knees in position but draw them slightly outward as if holding a balloon between them.

■ Keep your lower back straight by tilting your pelvis slightly up and forward. Avoid leaning backward because it can create tension in the hips.

■ Tuck your abdomen in slightly. Think of your pelvic area as a bowl holding your organs up.

■ Loosen your chest. This provides more room for your heart and lungs and makes them more "comfortable." This, in turn, slows the heart rate and calms the breathing, allowing yin (earth) energy to come up from the feet through the legs and into your torso and then pass through the insides of your arms and out your hands.

■ Round your upper back slightly, keep your shoulders even, open, and relaxed.

- Form a circle with your arms, keeping them far enough from the torso so that there is a space under the armpits. This space is created by holding the elbows wide apart and not allowing your shoulders to rise. It is as if there were a pillow beneath your torso and your arms.
- Make sure your hands are far enough apart that the qi has room to move. Relax your wrists. Bent wrists cut off qi flow to fingers.
- Relax your chin. If you hold your chin too high, this stops the spine from being straight and creates shoulder tension.
- Remember to touch your tongue lightly to your upper palate with your mouth softly closed.
- Keep your lower jaw and facial muscles relaxed.
- Keep your eyes level and relax the muscles between them. Look out into the distance with a soft focus. This creates a state the Chinese sages called shen yi qi, which translates as "spirit mind energy." As you look out into the distance, your spirit, intention, and vital energy are expressed simultaneously through your eyes, and these three components merge together. Where you look is where you direct your qi, so do not focus on a particular object but rather at a clear spot in the distance. If there is an obstruction in your line of vision, such as a wall, simply look through it.

To reap the benefits of the posture, it is essential to align your center while practicing Standing Like a Tree.

Practice each posture one after the other as described below. After you get to know the postures better, you may select one or more of your favorites to practice for an extended period of time.

STANDING POSITION 1: Extend your arms out in front of your middle *dantian,* with your arms rounded in toward your body. Bend your wrists at a forty-five-degree angle with your palms facing your heart, keeping your fingers spread. Your palms may tingle as the qi flows into them. Your shoulders are relaxed and your buttocks tucked under. Imagine yourself as a tree, with all the strength and separateness that entails. You are connected to the world around you, but also completely independent. Feel that sense of inner strength increasing as you stand.

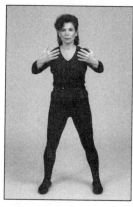
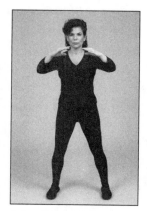
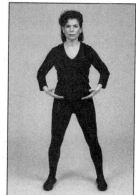

● *Standing Position 1* ● *Standing Position 2* ● *Standing Position 3*

STANDING POSITION 2: Maintain the same static posture as in standing position 1 but turn your palms down as if your arms are resting on the top half of a big qi ball. Experience the buoyant sense of energy flowing within the imaginary ball. Feel your body expand when you inhale and contract when you exhale. Breathe naturally and concentrate on your *dantian* as usual, and as you do so, notice the gentle expansion and contraction that occurs with the entire body.

STANDING POSITION 3: Move your hands out around the front of the big qi ball from standing position 2 and bring them down to rest at the level of your lower *dantian*. With your palms facing upward, notice a feeling of heaviness as you hold the imaginary qi ball. You may have a dense sensation on the backs of your hands and your palms may feel light and tingly, absorbing energy from the ball.

STANDING POSITION 4: From standing position 3, turn your palms downward toward the ground. There will be a pulling sensation on both the tops of your wrists and in your palms as your hands experience the energy of the ball above and the earth below. Notice the qi radiating from the earth into your palms. Look out into the distance and allow an overall sense of calm and peace to fill your entire being.

STANDING POSITION 5: Move your hands up the outside of the big qi ball from standing position 4, until they are an inch above your eyebrows.

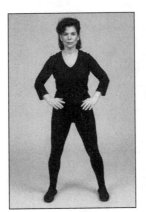
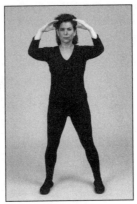
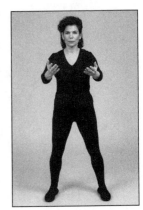

● *Standing Position 4*　　　● *Standing Position 5*　　　● *Standing Position 6*

Turn your palms downward and look out to the horizon. You may experience tingling in your hands and throughout your whole body as your arms round the top of the ball.

STANDING POSITION 6: Move your hands down and around the sides of the large qi ball, until you are holding its bottom sides. Extend your fingertips out in front of you with your palms facing upward, your hands relaxed, and with a rounded posture to your arms. Your elbows are slightly bent. Think about the energy of your heart as it promotes the free flow of blood throughout your body. Your tingling fingertips connect you to the outside world, catching qi from the heavens. Your hands may feel quite heavy, but your whole body is energized.

STANDING POSITION 7: This standing posture is exactly the same as standing position 6 except that the palms are turned downward. Experience the qi emanating from your fingertips. Feel a sense of tingling and warmth in your palms.

STANDING POSITION 8: Move your hands out to your sides and down to the height of your hips. Your palms face each other and rest about three feet apart as if you were picking up a huge tree stump. Feel the mixing of energy moving between your hands as a thick, invisible cord connects them. Your fingertips point down and there is an archlike bend in your arms. In this position, your qi forms an internal structure, supporting buoyancy, self-reliance, and a sense of inner protection.

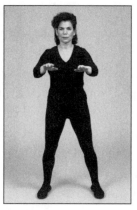
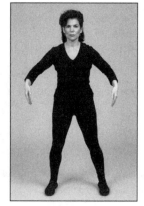

● *Standing Position 7*   ● *Standing Position 8*

Practice postures taking deep, rhythmic breaths for the duration of the exercise.

❀ Walking Like a Turtle *(1 minute)*

The arm positions of the eight different standing postures described above are also used in Walking Like a Turtle. Decide which of the eight positions you prefer. Hold your arms in that static position as you Walk Like a Turtle.

The walking exercise involves forward and backward movement. During both, your movement is slow and focused. Concentrate your mind on the bottoms of your feet as you relax your entire body to maintain proper balance. Keep your knees moderately bent and your body at the same height throughout the walking exercise. Relax your shoulders. Make sure to turn at the waist as you step out, lead with your waist. Remember that vision and focus follow the direction of your hands. Without moving your neck, imagine that the impulse for the movement comes from your forehead.

As you move, maintain the energy you developed while standing, keeping centered and connected along your front and back and your sides. Hold your physical "structure" intact as you move, not wavering. As you shift from side to side, your body remains an integrated whole. In order to maintain your integrity, move slowly. Don't let the energy you have gathered in the standing meditation seep out of you. This walking meditation helps you maintain your power as you move in the world.

Walking Forward Movement

Start in a standing position with your feet together, your weight distributed evenly on both legs, and your hands in the Standing Like a Tree posture of your choice. To begin your first step, shift your weight to your right leg, pick up your left foot and place it out in front of you, and circle it outward to the left of you, tracing the shape of a **C** or crescent. As you circle your foot to the left, hold your foot close to but not touching the ground in front of you. Next, shift most of your weight onto your left leg . Pick up your right foot and, keeping it close to the ground, draw it in toward your left foot. This completes your first step.

To begin your second step, circle the right foot out in front of you as you hold it close to but not touching the ground. Place your right foot down to the front and right of you. Maintain most of your weight on your left leg as you

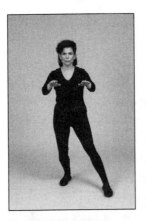
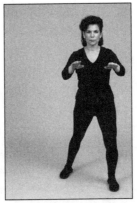
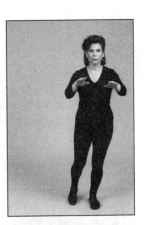

● *Walking Forward with Left Foot*

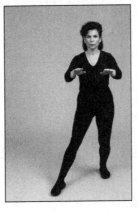
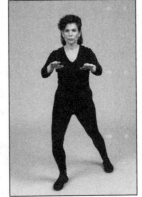
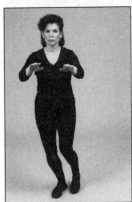

● *Walking Forward with Right Foot*

do this. Next, shift most of your weight onto your right leg. Bring your left foot in toward your right foot, holding it close to but not touching the ground. Finish your second step by shifting most but not all of your weight onto your right foot and leg.

Repeat the pattern of these steps as you walk forward, shifting your weight from one foot to the other. Your body remains at the same height the whole time, your buttocks tucked under. Your back is straight. Inhale as your foot moves toward the body and exhale as your foot moves away from the body. Walk forward six steps.

Walking Backward Movement

The backward steps are done in exactly the same pattern as the forward steps, but in reverse.

A complete Walking Like a Turtle exercise includes both forward and backward walking. After walking six steps forward, move straight into the backward movement, tracing six steps in reverse.

Take a total of twelve steps and a total of twelve complete breaths.

VARIATION ‖ When you become more accustomed to Walking Like a Turtle, move your arms in a rolling, circular fashion toward and then away from you in coordination with your breath and legs. Imagine there is a large ball in front of you. Breathe in as your foot lifts up and comes in toward the other foot and move your hands under the bottom of the imaginary ball toward your body. Breathe out as your foot makes contact with the ground, moving your hands over the top of the ball away from your body.

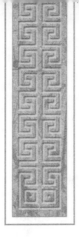

Set 5: Energize Endocrines

IN SET 5, we use our hands to send qi to our pituitary, hypothalamus, pineal, thyroid, parathyroid, thymus, pancreas, ovary, and adrenal glands. This promotes smooth functioning of these glands, which are catalysts for the proper functioning of all our bodily processes. These exercises are done without touching the body, by sending qi to your glands through *laogong,* and out the tips of your fingers (see illustration on page 20). How close your hands come to your body is an individual choice. Allow your movements to flow along with your imagination.

❀ Scooping Qi Posture

All of the following exercises begin with the Scooping Qi position. Stand comfortably with feet about a foot apart and hands at your sides. Begin your scooping motion by rounding your arms slightly and squatting lightly as if getting ready to sit on a chair, bending forward slightly at the waist. As you

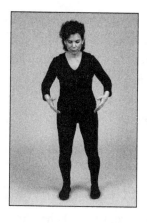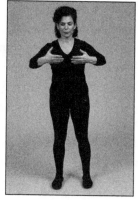

● *Scooping Qi*

squat, open your arms wide to each side of you at about hip level, with your palms facing each other and also wide apart. Move your arms down and gradually bring them to the center of your body. Keep your arms rounded as you move them down. Palms move toward one another in a gathering motion, fingertips pointing down as they descend toward the earth.

As you scoop qi from the earth, you may notice that your hands feel heavy. When you have gathered the qi, inhale, straighten at your waist and carry the qi upward toward the location of the endocrine gland you are focusing on. Your fingertips should be nearly touching as you move your rounded arms up the center of your body to chest level.

Do this scooping motion prior to sending qi to each of the glands.

✷ Pituitary, Hypothalamus, and Pineal Glands
(15 seconds)

Inhale as you scoop qi from the earth and bring it to just above the crown of your head. On your exhalation, slowly and purposefully wave your moderately tensed, vibrating hands, sending qi to your pituitary, hypothalamus, and pineal glands. All three of these endocrine glands are located in the center of the brain. Let your hands and mind linger over each gland individually if you need more time after the exhalation is complete.

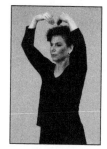

● *Pituitary, Hypothalamus, and Pineal Glands*

Silently thank the pituitary for its work as the "master gland" that helps many of your other glands function properly and regulates an entire range of bodily activities from growth to reproduction. Send good intent to your hypothalamus, which, as a part of the brain, connects the nervous system with the endocrine system, and as an endocrine gland has a direct effect on pituitary gland function. Give love and appreciation to your pineal gland for retarding the aging process, regulating menstruation and ovarian hormone secretion, and promoting normal brain function.

Practice once for a total of one complete breath.

✿ Thyroid and Parathyroid Glands *(12 seconds)*

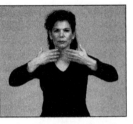

● *Thyroid and Parathyroid Glands*

Hold your neck erect and centered, but not stiff. Inhale and gather qi from the earth and then bring it up to the front of your neck. Exhale and emit qi from your hands, sending vital energy to your thyroid. Thank your thyroid for maintaining healthy organ function and optimal metabolism for you. Focus attention on your four parathyroid glands, located next to the lobes of the thyroid. Silently express appreciation for their help in maintaining your calcium and phosphorous levels, which support strong bones.

Practice once for a total of one complete breath.

✿ Thymus Gland *(12 seconds)*

Your thymus gland is located just above the midline of your breasts on your sternum area. Inhale, scooping qi from the earth and bringing your hands up to the area above your breasts. Exhale and send energy and kind thoughts to your thymus, thanking it for strengthening the immune system and keeping cells healthy. When finished, thump gently over your sternum twelve times with a closed fist. As you thump, picture your thymus glowing with vibrant health.

Practice once for a total of one complete breath.

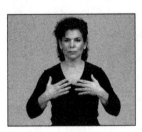
● *Thymus Gland*

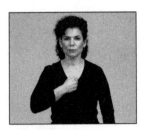
● *Thymus Thump*

VISUALIZATION ‖ As you thump your thymus, picture it glowing with vibrant health. See it vibrate with energy, ready to gobble up all obstacles in its way.

❀ Pancreas *(12 seconds)*

Inhale and gather qi from the earth. Exhale as you place your hands over the left side of your abdomen and concentrate your mind on your pancreas, fluttering your hands and sending it healing qi. Thank your pancreas for regulating your blood sugar levels, which allows for proper nourishment to your cells, and also thank it for promoting healthy digestion.

Practice once for a total of one complete breath.

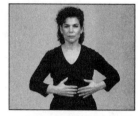

● *Pancreas Gland*

❀ Ovaries *(12 seconds)*

Inhale and gather qi from the earth. Breathe out as you place your hands over your lower abdomen close to your pubic bone. With your hands, send waves of energy to your ovaries, which have provided you with ripened eggs and flowing menses for many years. Thank your ovaries for this and ask that they continue to provide you with a healthy balance of sex hormones (estrogen, testosterone, progesterone) that brings a calm mind, restful sleep, healthy skin, strong bones and tissue, and vibrant sexual energy.

Practice once for a total of one complete breath.

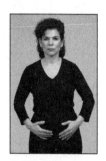

● *Ovary Glands*

❀ Adrenal Glands *(12 seconds)*

Gather qi from the earth as you inhale. Exhale and place your hands over your lower back near your kidneys and move them in a wavelike motion over this area. Think about how your two adrenal glands have helped you survive the stress in your life. Tell them how much you appreciate them now and promise to reduce stress in your life. Send your adrenal glands energy so they may continue to get you through stressful situations, help your immune system function optimally, control electrolyte balance, balance cholesterol levels, maintain normal metabolism, promote bone density, and maintain healthy energy levels.

Practice once for a total of one complete breath.

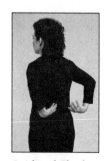

● *Adrenal Glands*

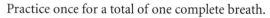

❁ Energize Endocrines Finale *(15 seconds)*

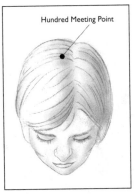

Hundred Meeting Point

● *Hundred Meeting Point*

Stand or sit comfortably with your hands relaxed at your sides or on your belly. Concentrate on the Hundred Meeting point at the very top of your head. Bring vibrant healing energy into this point from above and allow it to flow down through your body. Visualize your pituitary, hypothalamus, pineal, thyroid, parathyroid, thymus, pancreas, ovaries, and adrenals bathed and immersed in this energy. When you are ready, send this energy now to your *dantian* and store it there. Enjoy any sensations of calm and peace you experience.

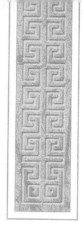

Set 6: Knitting Strong Bones

3 MINUTES 40 SECONDS

THIS set begins with weight-bearing exercises using qi balls for strengthening bones. It goes on to include Bone Marrow Washing exercises created to cleanse and nourish your bones, one of the most important parts of the body to care for as we age. Using qi balls stimulates the body physically through lifting weights in conjunction with qigong movements. With Bone Marrow Washing, mental imagery is combined with physical movements as you access your reservoirs of qi.

🏵 Playing Qi Ball (2 minutes)

Many of the exercises I describe throughout the workout can be adapted to accommodate weighted qi balls. These are specially designed balls of varying weights that improve the flow of energy and provide the weight-bearing benefit of strengthening bones. The exercises below illustrate and explain specifically how to use the balls, which can be found in a variety of health and fitness stores. If you don't have qi balls, you can use hand weights of one to five pounds in each hand or improvise with other weighted objects of your choice.

All movements in Playing Qi Ball stem from the waist. Throughout these movements, gently bend your knees. As you rotate the qi balls, shift from one foot to your center, and then to the other foot. This enables your arms to follow the movement of your waist rather than vice versa.

Throughout the movements, concentrate your attention on *laogong,* the center point of your palms. Holding weights in your hands can help you to be more conscious of this point. You may notice a heavy, dense sensation in the center of your palm. Notice the tips of your fingers filling with qi, too.

Keep your eyes focused on the balls as they move out in front of you. When you carry your qi balls upward, imagine you are bringing up qi from the earth. As you bring your qi balls downward, imagine you are bringing down qi from the heavens. Then mix the energies of the heaven and earth within yourself.

Lifting Qi Ball *(30 seconds)*

Stand with your feet together with a ball in each hand. Your hands rest by your hips, your elbows pointing behind you. In this exercise, you alternate between lifting the ball in your right hand and lifting the ball in your left hand.

Inhale and, with slightly bent elbow, bring the ball in your right hand forward and diagonally up and across your body, ending in a gesture of offering as you complete the inhalation with your hand at shoulder level. At the same time, your left hand flexes back in the opposite direction and you draw the

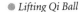
● *Lifting Qi Ball*

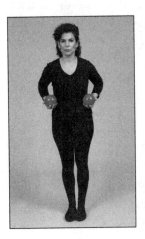
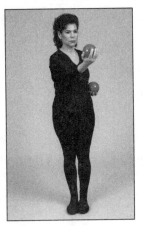
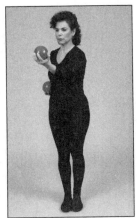

other ball back behind your left side. Gently twist to the left as you move your arm.

Next, exhale and repeat the movement. Bring your right hand back until it is at your side. Move the ball in your left hand forward and diagonally up and across your body.

Move slowly and keep your eyes fixed on the hand holding the qi ball as it extends out in front of you. Notice a subtle opening of your chest and the lengthening of your spine.

Repeat the cycle three times, for a total of three complete breaths.

As you breathe, be aware of the health of your breasts and the tremendous opening in your chest. The longer and slower your movements, the heavier the qi balls become. Go slowly, enjoying the push-and-pull motion of qi as you move, the hand moving backward becoming light, representing yin, as the one moving forward becomes heavy, representing yang.

Spinning Wheel *(45 seconds)*

Stand with your feet slightly wider apart than your shoulders, feet parallel, and knees slightly bent. Hold a ball in each hand, hands resting in front of your *dantian.* Holding them level and next to each other, move the balls in one big, clockwise circle. Shift your weight and move your arms first to the left, next up over your head, next to the right, and then back to center in the starting position, hands in front of your *dantian.* Inhale when moving across the bottom of the circle, exhale when moving over the top.

● *Spinning Wheel*

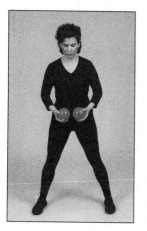
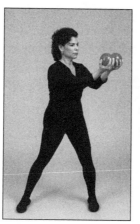
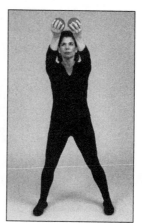
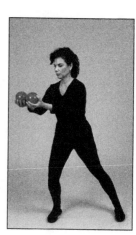

All movements in this exercise stem from the waist. Gently bend your knees. As your qi balls rotate, shift your weight from one foot, to your center, and then to the other foot. This enables your arms to follow the movement of your waist rather than vice versa. Concentrate on the balls with your eyes. Notice them get very heavy as you extend your arms, heavy above your head, less heavy at the side, and heaviest as you lower them.

This movement brings great awareness of the present moment, while also connecting you to the circular motion of time as your hands move around the "clock," through hours, days, seasons, and years. Notice the difference in sensation when you change direction.

Practice this exercise two times in each direction, first clockwise and then counterclockwise for a total of four complete breaths.

Back Swinging Monkey (45 seconds)

Stand with your feet together. Holding a ball in each hand, rest your hands in front of your *dantian*. Lower your arms to your sides, then opening them wide and turning to the left without moving your feet, swing your right arm forward and the left backward. Both balls follow an arc and end up at shoulder height, one in front of you and the other in back. Next, drop the balls simultaneously to your sides, turning to the right without moving your feet. Repeat this movement on the other side.

Inhale as the balls move upward and exhale as they swing downward. Follow the ball moving behind you with your eyes as you twist at the waist. For the first time in the workout, you are becoming aware of what's behind you, "watching your own back" and getting a great stretch as you do. Initiate all

● *Back Swinging Monkey*

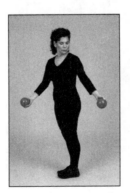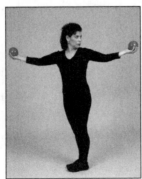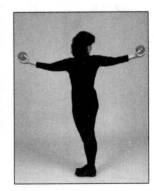

movements from the waist and be sure to lift your hands a little higher than your shoulders. At the height of the movement your chest is open to one side. This is also a great neck stretch as you look to the left and then the right. Think of youself twisting around the central axis that maintains your alignment.

As you switch positions, there is a subtle turn of the wrists. Keep your mind focused on *laogong* on the center of your palm and imagine a constant connection of qi between both your palms as you swing your qi balls to and fro. Remember the Bubbling Well point at the bottom of your feet, too, as you stretch tall.

Alternate from side to side.

Practice on each side three times for a total of six complete breaths.

❀ Bone Marrow Washing *(1 minute 40 seconds)*

You can do this exercise standing, sitting, or lying down. The following is a description of the standing position. This exercise is similar to Set 5: Energize Endocrines, where you use the qi accumulated in your body and send it to your bones through *laogong* and/or your fingertips. Take soft, slow, deep breaths as you nourish and purify your bones with earthly water and heavenly fire.

Bringing in Earthly Waters *(45 seconds)*

Begin by standing comfortably with your feet shoulder-width apart, knees slightly bent. As you inhale, bend over from the waist and scoop your hands toward the earth. Imagine you are scooping water from rivers, lakes, streams, and oceans up from the earth and into your body through the Bubbling Well point.

Next, continuing your inhalation, move your hands over your feet and ankles and imagine the water penetrating through these bone structures. Continue to move your hands up along your legs, the water nourishing the bones in your lower legs, your knees, and your thighs. Continue the same mental imagery as your hands move up to your abdominal area. Allow water to invigorate the structure of all the bones in this area, including your tailbone, sacrum, pelvis, and hip joints.

Next, move your hands up your torso as you concentrate the water in your lower, middle, and upper spine and rib cage. Complete your inhalation. Exhale as you move your hands over your collarbones, shoulder joints, down the inside of one arm and into your wrist and finger joints. Inhale as your hand moves back up the outside of your arm to the shoulder joints once again. Bathe the bones in this part of your body in the nourishing water from the earth. Repeat this pattern on the other side.

Take another exhalation and move your hands over your neck and up into the bones of your jaw, your teeth, then your skull. Imagine you are penetrating and invigorating these bone structures with healing water from the earth.

When you reach the top of the head, take a moment to experience the healing water gathering as you take a deep inhalation. Upon exhalation, drape your entire skeleton with imaginary water as if you were standing under a

● *Bringing in Earthly Waters*

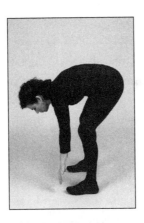
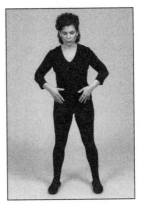
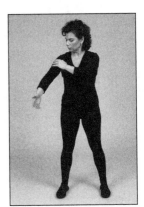
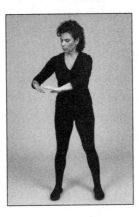
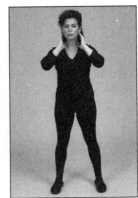
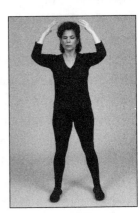

waterfall. Follow the flow of this imaginary water with your hands, moving from the top of your head to the tips of your toes and back into the earth through the Bubbling Well point.

Take four complete breaths as you do this exercise.

Bringing in Heavenly Fire (45 *seconds*)

Stand comfortably with your feet shoulder-width apart, knees slightly bent. As you inhale, raise your arms and bring the fire from the sun and stars down into your head through your Hundred Meeting point and down to your upper spine. Using your hands, exhale and move the imaginary fire down the inside of one arm and inhale as you move it up the outside of the same arm. Repeat sides, exhaling then inhaling. Exhale as you continue down your spine to your feet, visualizing fire penetrating your body as it passes downward and into the Bubbling Well point on each foot.

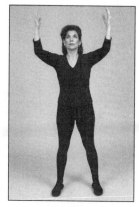

● *Bringing in Heavenly Fire*

Inhale and experience the healing fire gathered throughout your body. Exhale and visualize heavenly fire penetrating, nourishing, and purifying your entire skeleton. Following the flames back up with your hands, moving from the tips of your toes up to the top of your head, send the fire back into the heavens where it originated.

Take four complete breaths as you do this exercise.

❁ Mixing Fire and Water (*10 seconds*)

After completing both visualizations, hold one hand over your middle *dantian* (representing fire) and the other over your lower *dantian* (representing water) as you consciously mix water and fire within your body. The parts of your body that have too much fire are soothed by the water. Those that have too much water are enlivened by the activation of the fire. After mixing, remember to send the fire back to the heavens and the water back to the earth.

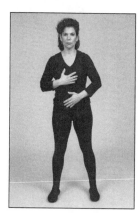

● *Mixing Water and Fire*

As you complete this exercise, notice how clean your body and mind feel. Notice the circulation of qi in your bones and in your brain. Qi is nourishing both and maintaining their proper function. The nourishment of your marrow has, in turn, nourished your vital organs, which has lit a spark in your spirit!

Practice for the duration of one to two deep breaths.

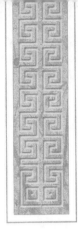

Set 7: Nourishing Three Treasures

THE QIGONG exercise in this set nourishes and balances your vital energy (qi), the essence of your bodily secretions (*jing*), and your connection to higher consciousness, or spirit (*shen*). These are known as the Three Treasures. In traditional Chinese medicine, how you cultivate and protect the Three Treasures determines the quality and length of your life. Perform this set with slow, purposeful movements and allow your treasures to shine from within.

❀ Lady Raises Lotus to the Temple *(2 minutes)*

Stand with your feet wider than shoulder-width apart, pointing out at a forty-five-degree angle. Keep your back straight, head erect, hands by your sides, and buttocks tucked under. Begin your inhalation and bend forward from your waist, reaching down with your hands. Bring energy into both of your hands as you scoop up an imaginary lotus flower from the ground.

Raise the flower upward along the center of the front of your body, first to your lower *dantian* and then up to the middle *dantian*. Notice any heaviness or tingling in your hands. In this upward motion, your arms are rounded, palms face up, fingertips point toward each other and almost touch, and there is a taut sensation in your palms. Notice the qi gathering in your fingertips. Complete your first inhalation as your hands arrive at the midline of your chest at the middle *dantian*. Elbows bent, your palms face upward on a horizontal plane across the front of your body.

On your exhalation, extend your hands out in front of you, pinky fingers touching. Feel the qi flowing out of the tips of your fingers as you extend your

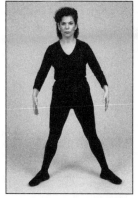

● *Lady Raises Lotus to the Temple Beginning Posture*

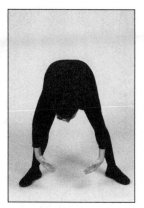

● *Gathering Lotus Flower*

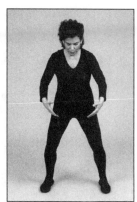

● *Nourishing Jing Treasure*

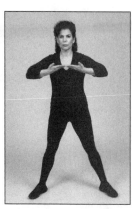

● *Nourishing Qi Treasure*

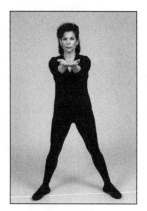

● *Offering Lotus Flower*

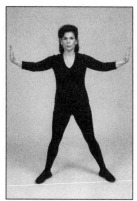

● *Arms Open Wide, Palms Pushing Outward*

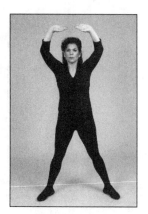

● *Nourishing Shen Treasure*

hands with elbows slightly bent. With your arms fully extended, your exhalation is complete as you offer your lotus flower to the world, your palms taut with qi.

Inhale and open your arms out wide at shoulder height, maintaining a slight bend in your elbows. Continue until your arms extend out, palms still facing up as you complete your inhalation.

Next, arms still lifted, exhale and push your palms out as if you are pushing against imaginary walls to each side of you. Imagine that you are expelling all of the negative energy from your body as you exhale and push out with your palms. Again, your palms are as taut as the skin of a drum. Imagine cords

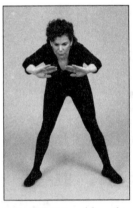
● *Bending Forward from the Waist*

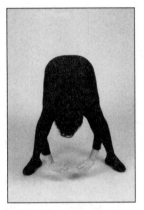
● *Palms Facing the Earth*

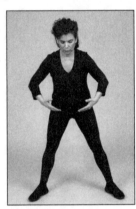
● *Nourishing Jing Treasure*

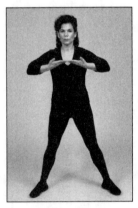
● *Nourishing Qi Treasure*

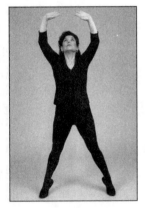
● *Nourishing Shen Treasure*

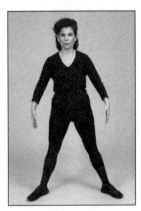
● *Lady Raises Lotus to the Temple Ending Posture*

of qi streaming out of them up from your lower and middle *dantian*. This motion creates a tremendous amount of female power.

Inhale and begin raising your hands up toward the sky, palms still facing out, fingertips leading as your arms form an arc above you. At the end of this movement, your fingertips point toward each other, palms pushing up toward the sky. Your entire being is full of *shen*, as you experience lightness and clarity. This stimulates your upper *dantian*, the reservoir of spiritual energy located just above the point at the center of your eyes.

Begin your exhalation and bend forward from your waist, arms extending in a rounded position in front of you, pushing your palms outward and downward. Finish your exhalation with your back straight, palms facing the earth and hands filled with heaviness again.

Inhale and fan your fingertips out. Scoop the qi, lifting the flower up again along the front and center of your body. Fingertips touch at your middle *dantian*. Push your palms up as you continue on toward the heavens and lift up onto your toes. Again, you experience a sensation of great female power and a burst of energy. Begin the last exhalation, opening your arms out to your sides with palms facing down, fingertips trailing behind, and arms outstretched. Allow your hands to flow gently down like leaves falling from a tree. End with your hands totally relaxed by your sides as you complete your exhalation.

Throughout this exercise keep your body aligned. Relax completely and imagine all the impurities leaving through your feet.

Practice three times, for a total of twelve complete breaths.

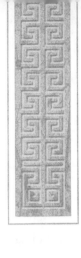

Warm-Down: Closing the Circle

THE WARM-DOWN gathers qi inward, consolidates it into a small ball and stores it within the lower *dantian,* your center of physical healing. This storehouse of qi can then be used sparingly, as needed. Each time you practice qigong you cultivate and add more qi riches to your *dantian,* the precious reservoir of healing vital energy. This is the area where your kidney essence *(jing)* resides. It is the birthplace of your life force and every woman's breeding ground for sexual growth, conception, reproduction, and menstruation. Proper growth and development in this area not only determines the quantity and quality of your life, but also the state of your emotions and spiritual enhancement. This final set promotes a life filled with energy, health, peace, and happiness.

❀ Mini Yin Massage *(15 seconds)*

Standing comfortably with your feet about a foot apart, gently massage your whole body. Beginning with one hand, knead the fingers on the opposite hand, then your palm, arm, and shoulder. Switch sides and repeat. Using both hands, massage your neck, the backs of both shoulders, and your scalp. Massage over your ribs and along both sides of your body, down the front of your legs and up again, along the backs of your legs. Notice where your tension is kept and work your muscles like dough, pressing and squeezing so deeply you can feel your bones.

NOTE ‖ Massage your legs and arms in a circular motion with the thumbs and tips of your fingers or the palm of the hand moving toward the joints and massaging around them. Always massage toward your heart center. Keep your entire hand open so that you can transmit qi to yourself more easily.

Self-massage can benefit nerve problems, but if you have severe inflammation of the nerves or an infectious disease, do not overdo it. Instead, stroke gently and lightly, avoiding deep pressure.

✹ Feathering *(10 seconds)*

Smooth the qi throughout your body by whisking yourself as if your fingers were feathers. Start first at the Hundred Meeting point at the crown of your head, and feather down the sides of your head and face and down the sides of your neck. Smooth the qi on each arm, using the opposite hand. Lightly brush one hand after another as if they are feathers down your neck and down the center of your torso. Do both legs and end at your toes. The sensation here is a gentle one, as if you are brushing yourself with kindness.

Do for up to ten seconds.

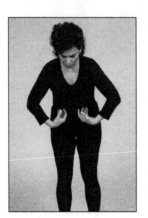
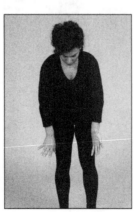

● *Feathering*

✿ Drinking Divine Water *(25 seconds)*

As you begin this exercise, visualize condensing the qi in your *dantian* into a small ball. Begin clicking your teeth vigorously and rapidly, but as lightly as possible with your mouth closed. You will hear the teeth clicking and feel a pleasurable vibration throughout your head. Click about thirty-six times.

With your mouth closed, roll your tongue around the outside of your teeth and gums in a clockwise circle. Then run your tongue along the inside of your teeth and gums in a counterclockwise circle. Repeat this wonderful mouth massage in each direction three times.

You should now have a mouthful of saliva. Another way to think about this is that your mouth has filled with the water of life.

Swallow this vital water in one noisy gulp. Let the healing water your body has created wash and moisten your internal organs. With your mind's eye, follow the path of the saliva downward to your *dantian*. Visualize the saliva turning into steam in your *dantian*. This is the qi that promotes healthy longevity.

✿ Smoothing Belly Qi *(30 seconds)*

This exercise is done for the purpose of storing the qi cultivated throughout the workout within your body and can be done sitting, standing, or lying down.

● *Storing Body Qi*

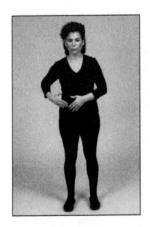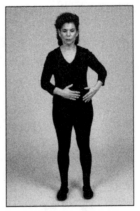

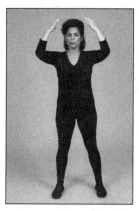
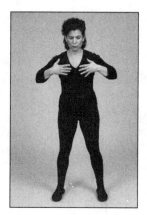
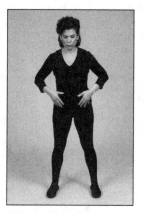
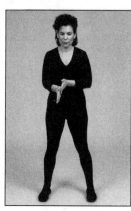

● *Connect with Upper Dantian* ● *Connect with Middle Dantian* ● *Connect with Lower Dantian* ● *Consolidate Your Qi*

If standing, keep your feet apart and your hands in front of your upper *dantian.* Palms face your body, fingertips are pointed toward each other, and arms are rounded.

If sitting, do so with your feet flat on the floor, back straight and head erect. If lying down, find a comfortable, soft surface. Make sure your head is in line with the rest of your body and that you are lying straight, your hips aligned with the rest of you.

Take a moment to connect with your *dantian.* Breathing naturally, place your hands over your lower *dantian* and move them around in a circle either above or actually touching your belly. Visualize the steam just created from Drinking the Divine Water condensing along with the qi into a small ball of energy to be stored in your *dantian.* Reverse the direction of your hands and continue the visualization.

Finally, take a moment to close the circle of energy you have activated during your workout by connecting with your upper, middle, and lower *dantians.* Place your hands over each *dantian* one after the other with your hands about two inches away from your body and your palms facing you. Relax your entire body. Concentrate your mind on your upper *dantian,* then your middle *dantian,* and lastly your lower *dantian.* Allow yourself to experience whatever sensations the qigong workout has given you. Notice the vital energy in and around you as you do so and create a protective shield around yourself. When you feel ready, drop your hands to a relaxed position by your sides.

Experience the sensation of total relaxation, noticing different feelings through-out your body.

Rub your hands together quickly until friction and heat are produced. This consolidates your qi, creating more energy for the next time you practice.

Your Twenty-Minute Workout is now complete.

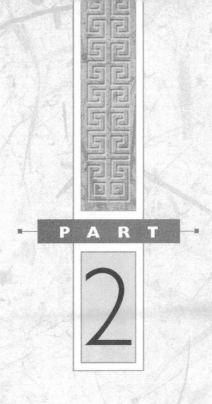

Understanding the Twenty-Minute Workout

The body should be supple like an infant
The movements should be flexible like a snake
The feeling should be soft like water
The breathing should be smooth like a cloud

QIGONG PROVERB

WHEN I began practicing qigong nearly thirty years ago, I learned first by doing, not by reading about qigong in books. It was not until after the movements had become second nature to me that I began to study the finer points of the practice and to understand some of the profound ideas behind the exercises. *Qigong for Staying Young* is designed so that you can have a similar experience.

In Part One, you learned the movements of the Twenty-Minute Workout. Here in Part Two, I explain the benefits of the movements and how to refine and deepen your practice. In the process, I provide a basic introduction to some of the ancient, nature-based concepts of Chinese medical philosophy, ideas that form the foundation of qigong.

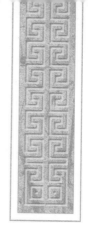

Body, Breath, and Mind

IN QIGONG, we learn to regulate our bodies, our breath, and our minds—a simple practice that can have wide-reaching impact in our lives. With regulation of the body, you learn to adjust your posture, relax, and develop strong "roots" to the earth. Regulation of the breath means you concentrate on your breathing. With each breath, you gather, stimulate, and circulate vital energy throughout your body. Your breathing becomes slow, gentle, rhythmic, and deep. Regulation of the mind helps you shed extraneous thoughts and focus your awareness on particular parts of your body.

The position of your body creates the base from which you move. Your breath activates the qi flow and your mind guides the qi where it needs to go.

As you become more adept at the movements in the workout, they will become second nature to you. Your mind will become relaxed and you will experience the true essence and joy of qigong. In Chinese this qigong state is called *wang* or "no-mindedness." No-mindedness is a meditative state of being half-awake and half-forgetful, but in a good way!

REGULATION OF THE BODY

Most of the exercises in this book are performed in a standing or walking position, but they can all be adapted based upon individual needs. You may also choose to sit or lie down for any part of the workout, the warm-up included. No matter what your position, if your body is properly aligned you will experience a smooth flow of qi, regular and rhythmic breathing, and a relaxed state of mind. The following explanations of posture apply to general movements in the set. Specific exercises vary.

When Sitting or Lying Down

Sit down comfortably on the front of a chair. Rest your feet flat on the floor and your hands palms down on your lap. Check that your back is straight and your chin is relaxed. If your feet don't reach the floor—as mine sometimes don't—you can place a phone book, a pillow, or some other leveling object under them.

If you prefer to lie down, lie on your back with your legs extended, your feet shoulder-width apart. If you prefer to keep your knees raised, prop them up with a pillow. This helps take the strain off your back. Allow your hands to rest comfortably at your sides or on your belly.

People who are unable to walk or are physically challenged often do qigong exercises in these positions. Whatever your physical abilities, you can adapt most qigong exercises to achieve the same potent healing results.

When Standing

What surface should I practice on?

Practice on any surface including indoor flooring, an outdoor hard surface like asphalt, a wooden deck, a sandy beach, or a grassy field. When you practice qigong on these different surfaces, notice the difference in the way your qi is flowing. I have led classes on every surface from tennis courts to lawns. Sometimes a hard outdoor surface helps us focus better because we don't have to worry about sogginess, lumps, or bumps. A grassy area or a sandy beach gently stimulates us with nature's own energy. If you experience problems with balance, it is best to practice on a flatter surface. Choose the surface that works best for you.

How should I position my feet?

Foot positions vary with each posture but no matter what the position of your feet, make sure that your soles are relaxed. Take a minute to concentrate on each toe, then on the front, middle, and back of your feet. As you relax your soles, you'll notice that your entire body relaxes, too. You will also feel more connected to the earth, experiencing a rooted sensation that supports your whole body.

What about my knees?

Don't lock your knees. Keep them slightly bent to remain steady and grounded to the earth. When a posture calls for deep bending, the more deeply you bend your knees, the stronger you will feel and the more your qi will flow. This is because a lower center of gravity provides a better base of support and connection to the earth. Don't sacrifice good form, however—bend your knees only as deeply as you can while still maintaining proper alignment.

What position is best for my head and neck?

Hold your head and neck in a natural but upright position. Imagine a golden thread suspending your body from above at the very top of your head. Relax your neck. This allows the free flow of blood and qi between head and body.

Where should I focus my eyes?

In general, focus your eyes either straight out or slightly down in front of you into the distance. This ensures that your qi stays focused, too, helping you to move the qi wherever you want it to go. Your eyelids can be relaxed and open or slightly closed.

How about my mouth and tongue?

Practice with a closed mouth so you can breathe in and out through your nose. This warms and cleanses the inhaled air and stimulates nasal nerve endings to enhance bodily functions such as heart rate, blood pressure, and respiration. Keep your lips gently pursed, your lower jaw relaxed and slightly drawn in toward your neck. This creates a better circulation of qi around the three *dantians*.

Rest your tongue on the roof of your mouth just behind the front of your teeth, creating a conduit for the qi to circulate throughout your system.

If there is an increase in saliva in your mouth while you practice, don't spit it out. Instead swallow it slowly in one big gulp. This benefits your digestion and nurtures your organ systems.

What about my chin?

Keep your chin tilted downward slightly. This helps you maintain a flat, straight upper back. Pointing the chin up breaks the natural flow of qi and constricts the qi moving upward along the spine.

How should my shoulders be held?

Relax your shoulders and let arms hang naturally. Relaxed shoulders promote proper qi flow from the neck down through the arms and into the hands.

How about my back?

Maintain a relaxed, flat back. Leaning backward or forward during your practice limits the amount of qi flowing up the spine, adversely affecting the overall health of the body. When you keep your back straight, you can gather qi from heaven and earth and allow a natural flow so you don't lose energy or get tired. Bending forward or backward also suppresses lung qi and can lead to shortness of breath. As you practice, draw your chest and abdomen in slightly to keep your back straight. Do not hunch your shoulders. Relax your hips and tuck your buttocks under so that the qi circulates up the center of your back.

How should I hold my arms?

As you move through the movements, bend your elbows slightly and imagine a pillow between your arms and your sides.

What about my wrists and fingers?

Relax your wrists. Keep your fingers loose, slightly bent, and naturally spread. This posture encourages the flow of qi up your arms and throughout your body during the qigong workout.

OTHER TIPS ‖ It can be extremely helpful to practice your qigong in front of a mirror to check the position of your body.

Practice far away from pollution, fumes, traffic, and so on. Turn off the TV and radio, as excess noise can disrupt the rhythm and flow of qi. Many people enjoy practicing to gentle, flowing music. I prefer finding music in silence.

Ready the body to create a solid base from which to move. Each posture facilitates a unique pattern of qi flow in the body. For example:

- Upward body movements raise qi.
- Downward body movements sink qi.
- Opening movements disperse qi outward.
- Closing movements gather qi inward.

At the same time qi flows within a certain body part, it is flowing between parts as you move. For this reason, practice the movements just as they are described and shown.

REGULATION OF THE BREATH

Regulation of the breath teaches you to alter quantity and quality of the breath and the duration of inhalation and exhalation. With qigong breathing, you take in a maximum amount of air with a minimum amount of effort. This also helps you direct qi to various areas of your body, giving these areas a breath of fresh air both literally and figuratively. Regular, rhythmic, and full breathing strengthens lung and heart function, promotes more efficient exchange of oxygen and carbon dioxide, keeps the blood pure and the brain nourished, and calms the mind. Qigong breathing soon becomes part of your everyday life. When you are aware of your breath, you will be more "in the moment." You may even find yourself using deep breathing when you are not practicing qigong to help you through stressful situations.

Qigong breathing is different from the way people normally breathe in our society. Many Western adults have adopted tight abdominal muscles and the bad habit of holding their chests high, which creates shallow breathing. Watch babies on the other hand and you will notice they naturally breathe qigong style. Qigong masters, like babies, maintain relaxed, soft bellies as they breathe. This promotes good qi flow, fabulous health, and a beautiful, youthful appearance.

The coordination of your breathing and your movements creates a particular effect on the body. For example, inhaling raises and contracts the flow of qi while exhaling sinks and expands qi flow. In general, when you are doing rising movements, inhale, and when doing sinking movements, exhale. When moving to the left and right, inhale or exhale naturally. Initially, you will need to concentrate on this new way of breathing, but in time you will do it without even thinking.

Throughout some of the workout, you simply breathe naturally, rhythmically, and deeply, coordinating breath with your movement without thinking too much about it. At other times, I ask you to pay special attention to breathing deeply with the movement, really expanding your abdomen upon inhalation and contracting it upon exhalation. At these times, imagine the air coming into your belly and blowing it up like a balloon on inhalation, and deflating the balloon on exhalation. This technique stimulates qi flow within the *dantian.*

When you breath in, imagine the air (also known as qi) coming in from the outside through your nose, down your throat, down to your chest, into your lungs, down to your abdomen, and into your *dantian.* When you exhale, visualize the air leaving your *dantian* and going back up to your chest and lungs, coming up your trachea, past your throat, up though your nasal passages, and out your nose.

Visualize vital and fresh energy flowing into your body upon inhalation. Visualize stagnant energy expelled from your body upon exhalation.

If you decide to expand your studies of qigong, you will find other, sometimes more advanced, breathing methods to learn. For our purposes here, it is enough to learn to breathe like a baby again!

REGULATION OF THE MIND

As you practice, free your mind of unnecessary distractions, concerns, and negative thoughts. This is not always easy. However, it is one of the most beneficial things you can do for yourself while practicing qigong. This practice is called training the mind to return to the void, another way of describing a qigong state. The more you can achieve this state, the more beneficial your qigong will be. Obsessive thoughts create blockages of qi that lead to chronic stagnation. To quiet your mind, concentrate on your movements and your breath.

As women, we too often find ourselves trapped by the way we relate to others. Whether it be our parents, significant other, children, friends, a boss or a co-worker, focusing too much on others and not enough on ourselves is detrimental to our emotional health. According to Chinese medicine emotional upset is often the root cause of our physical ailments. Qigong practice is a time for *us,* a time to clear our minds of all outer concerns and allow our personal qi, combined with the energy of the universe, to care for us.

Qigong calms us down, but do avoid practicing if you are feeling overly emotional. If your heart and mind are not tranquil, you won't be able to move your qi down into your lower *dantian* as easily. The qi accumulated in your lower *dantian* feeds into your other *dantian*s and is responsible for the physical health of your body and subsequent emotional and spiritual development. If you are upset and the only way you can calm yourself is to practice qigong, that's understandable, but please make this the exception, not the rule.

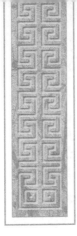

Flow of Qi

THE FIRST two sets in the workout open the overall flow of qi throughout your body. Stored in the *dantians,* qi travels through your body by way of meridians, invisible pathways for energy that run from the top of your head to the tips of your toes and also between your major organs. Though invisible, these pathways conduct energy much the way our circulatory or nervous systems conducts blood and electrical impulses.

Located along the main meridians are various acupoints, spots that, when stimulated, allow you to tap into deeper energies of the body and to direct and alter qi flow. Each acupoint (also known as an acupuncture or acupressure point) affects the body in a specific way. During your qigong practice, many meridians and their acupoints are stimulated, protecting and balancing the body. This stimulation provides ample vital energy and blood, nourishing the physical structures of your body so they maintain and sustain you for life.

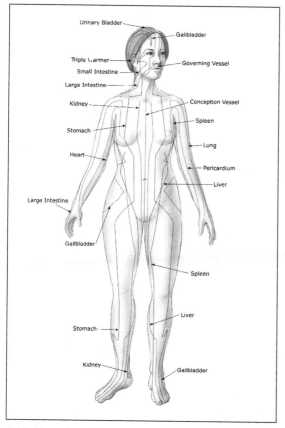

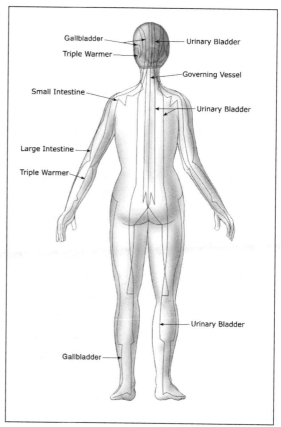

● *Meridians: Front View*

● *Meridians: Back View*

WARM UP: WAKING UP QI

A warm-up is an essential part of any exercise program, a wake-up call for your whole body, and especially for your body's qi. This warm-up is a well-rounded, enjoyable combination of exercises that, by moving qi, invigorates muscles and relaxes the spirit. All of the warm-up exercises promote flexibility and strength of the joints, muscles, tendons, and ligaments that will be working for you during your workout. The warm-up revitalizes the fluid that lubricates the joints, helping to prevent the pain that occurs when qi becomes stuck there. The qigong warm-up exercises also enhance the elasticity of your muscle tissue, helping maintain greater flexibility even after your workout is complete. When your muscles are elastic and well stretched, your ligaments and tendons are more stable. These exercises also moisten and nourish your tendons, allowing joints and muscles to move freely. This in turn prevents symptoms such as muscular weakness, spasms, contractions, impaired movement, and tremors. The warm-up helps prevent injury generally, both in and beyond your workout.

When you wake up your body qi, you also stimulate your brain. Yes, qigong will make you smarter! Each movement generates fluid flows that lubricates the spinal cord, regulates communication between nerves, and nourishes the mind.

The warm-up is generally performed at a quick pace and exercises your muscles. This means that, compared to the sets that follow in the Twenty-Minute Workout, the warm-up is a more *external* form of qigong. Sets 1 through 7 are more *internal* because they cultivate qi and blood. You will notice as you practice that the workout begins with external movements and gradually introduces internal practices such as visualization and sending qi to your organs, glands, and bones. This is because we must first have a strong physical body in order to develop ourselves internally.

As you do these exercises, the energy in your body begins to swirl. As you wake up this energy, you prepare your body and mind for the burst of energy to come, for the qi that will rebalance and reawaken all aspects of your being. Especially if you are practicing in the morning, the warm-up prepares you not only for the workout to follow but for the day ahead.

Mentally, this can be a time to remember and reflect on what yesterday held and to look forward to what today will bring. Release negative thoughts and feelings and fill yourself with clean, fresh energy. This will help you go forward, through the workout and into your day, whatever it has in store. As you apply qigong principles to your life goals, you will be surprised how many dreams come true.

Prepare yourself to begin your warm-up by quieting any mental "noise" you are experiencing. Envision unnecessary thoughts float away as if they are fluffy white clouds. Position your body, take a deep breath, and center yourself in the present moment. Become as centered and as relaxed as possible. As you do these movements, gently but purposefully thrust your energy forward and wake up your body and mind. Upon finishing, you may feel warmth in your fingertips, a brewing energy in your *dantian*, a tingling throughout your body, a heightened state of awareness, and a calm and focused state of mind.

Beautiful Woman Turns at Waist and Beautiful Woman Turns at Hips

In addition to strengthening the lower back, joints, and bones, and increasing flexibility, these two exercises enliven the important area around your lower *dantian*. This stimulates the kidneys, which are said to be the root of life, the very source of our vital energy.

Any qigong movement that stimulates the lower back, like these first two warm-ups, opens the flow of qi to the kidneys and thus affects aspects of you that relate to these organs. In Chinese medical philosophy, the kidneys are related to fear and worry. The health of the kidneys influences how you do things in life. Are you afraid to speak your mind, timid about new things? Do you sometimes allow fear and worry to stop you from living your life to the fullest? Do you know what you want and go for it? Practicing these qigong movements and others to strengthen kidney qi will help you take important chances in your life and overcome your fears.

Because the first exercise opens the waist, it circulates flow of qi around the lower *dantian* and *mingmen* point.

As you learned in Part One, the lower *dantian* is considered the physical center of healing and the center from which all movements stem. It is the area of the body that we focus on most in qigong, believed by the Chinese to be one of the first areas developed during the primary formation of our bodies in the womb.

Mingmen is an acupoint on your back, located directly behind the *dantian* between the kidneys and just beneath the spine, where all energy pathways related to physical health and well being are connected. *Mingmen* is extremely important. Formed at the moment of our conception, it is considered the center of transformations in our body's energy. Energy moves back and forth between the *dantian* and *mingmen*. These areas are so interconnected they are often thought of as one.

Both of these exercises help to alleviate lower back pain, pelvic pain, and gynecological problems. Beautiful Woman Turns at Hips in particular brings qi to your lower erogenous zones, which means you may feel sex-

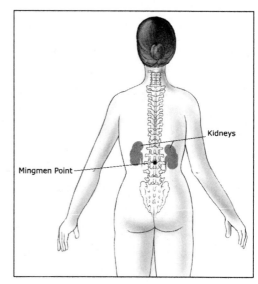

Kidneys

Mingmen Point

● *Mingmen Point*

ier than you have in a long while! Emotionally, both exercises help you maintain your own center and avoid overextending yourself with others.

Circling Knees

In addition to the benefits of the first two exercises, Circling Knees promotes qi circulation along the urinary bladder meridian, where the qi of the kidneys and many other organs is nourished.

Like the waist and hip circles, the knee circles not only stimulate qi flow to the kidneys but also the reflexology points on the bottom of the feet. These points are part of a microsystem in which treating an extremely small part of the body has the potential to heal the entire body. Tenderness on certain points on the soles of your feet relates to a particular part of the body. When you do these circular movements, you are stimulating points that open up the flow of energy throughout all systems and organs that may need attention.

Monkey Stretches Up and Down

This exercise continues to stimulate the kidneys and urinary bladder meridian and, in addition, promotes qi circulation in the lungs and heart. The coordination of movement with the breath, opening of the lower back, and the great upward stretch makes this exercise a favorite for many. It increases flexibility of the spine by stretching it in two complimentary yet opposite directions. Feel the variation of spinal sensation when you bring your hands downward versus upward. This up-and-down movement keeps the spaces between your vertebrae open and clear, allowing for maximum flow of nerve impulses along your spine.

Any qigong movement that expands and contracts the chest, like this one, opens the flow of qi to the lungs and thus affects aspects relating to the lungs. According to Chinese medical philosophy, the lungs are related to grief and depression, so don't be surprised if this exercise lifts your spirits.

The middle *dantian* is also stimulated during this exercise. This area of your body relates not only to how you experience your "space" but how you relate to others. Stimulating this area increases awareness about how you feel when you allow other people into your space and how you treat them once they are there.

When both of these areas of your body become opened through qigong, you will feel happier, release unresolved grief, and allow people to come into your life with greater ease. When you feel more whole, you will in turn treat others with graciousness and kindness and at the same time maintain healthy boundaries.

Opening Qi Door

Opening qi flow to your shoulders, arms, wrists, and hands is of utmost importance during the warm-up phase of the workout. When your shoulders and wrists are relaxed, qi and blood flow freely into your hands and fingertips, your instruments for self-healing. Later in the workout, you use the qi in your warm hands as a kind of healing balm for many other parts of your body.

This exercise and the following two exercises in the triad are done in the Horse Stance. Horse Stance, named for its similarity to the position you take when riding a horse, lowers the center of gravity below the *dantian,* which enhances your qi experience. Horse Stance replaces weakness in the legs with renewed strength and improves blood circulation, among other benefits.

Opening Qi Door will bring out the martial artist in you! Push the outer edge of your hands forward as if they were blades cutting through the air. Keep bad energy away from you by using those "blades" to protect yourself. This motion is not violent or aggressive, but comes from a stong heart.

Opening Qi Door opens both heart and lung meridians. Doing this exercise has an impact your interaction with others. You may notice changes in how you exchange love, how safe you feel, how much you trust that others can't hurt you, and the levels of jealousy and hate in your life. Practicing this exercise also helps you feel compassion and sympathy for others. When your heart and lungs are open and flowing with healthy qi, you feel love for yourself and embrace others in a soft, sweet, warm, and gentle way.

When you practice Opening Qi Door, you not only strengthen the qi in your lower *dantian* in Horse Stance, you embrace the special qi women know so well, the energy that springs from your heart and the middle *dantian.* Certain ancient practices that are specific to women focus primarily on the middle *dantian.* In this workout, although I include many exercises to enhance and open the energy of the heart, my focus is on helping you balance energies between all three energy centers in the body—the upper, middle, and lower *dantians.* While I honor the importance of the middle *dantian* for women, I see the lower *dantian* as the *fundamental* reservoir for healing in the body.

For both women and men, the lower *dantian* is the source on which our upper and middle *dantians* draw. Balance between all three energy centers is key.

Flapping Wrists

You may have noticed that you always feel colder than the males in your midst. Due to the predominantly cold nature of our bodies, women often have less blood flowing into the hands. The wrists are one of the most fragile joints in the body and are often slow to heal once injured. To help prevent injury, increase qi and blood flow to this area. Many of my students like to pretend they are waving at each other as they practice this movement. If you find yourself smiling at this naturally funny exercise, allow that smile to warm your entire being.

Separating Clouds

Separating Clouds balances yin and yang in the body. The concept of yin and yang has to do with the relationship of opposites. In nature and in our bodies, contrasting qualities such as passive and active, soft and hard, female and male, cold and hot, dark and light, or slow and fast engage in a subtle dance. Opposites complement each other, and every quality contains an element of its opposite. Yin always contains a little bit of yang and yang a little bit of yin.

When doing this movement, focus your mind on the *laogong* point at the center of each palm. Combined with the movement, concentrating on this

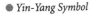
● *Yin-Yang Symbol*

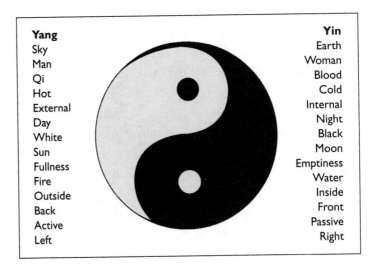

Yang	Yin
Sky	Earth
Man	Woman
Qi	Blood
Hot	Cold
External	Internal
Day	Night
White	Black
Sun	Moon
Fullness	Emptiness
Fire	Water
Outside	Inside
Back	Front
Active	Passive
Left	Right

point builds qi in your hands. As you raise your arms, imagine you are bringing yin energy up from the earth. As your arms descend, you are bringing yang energy down from the heavens. As your arms circle round and round, you mix yin and yang together, balancing energies perfectly.

When you do this exercise, you will experience a force propelling your arms around and around, so much so that they just move on their own. Feel free to also move your arms slowly if you prefer, inhaling as your arms rise and exhaling as they descend. Make sure that you relax your neck, shoulders, elbows, and wrists as you do this to unblock energy and allow it to flow through these areas. With each rotation, the expansive upward movement of the arms pumps blood to your heart and brain.

Separating Clouds also opens up the flow of qi in the shoulder joint by stimulating Large Intestine 15 (see illustration on page 157) on each shoulder, an area that is tense for many of us. With practice, qi flow increases and this area becomes softer, enhancing flexibility in the shoulders and arms. This point is also an important key in the regulation of women's hormones and is traditionally used for breast cancer prevention.

Brushing Wind

This simple exercise is wonderful for strengthening overall health and fitness because it opens qi and blood flow along a number of different meridians that come to an end in the hands. This movement extremely beneficial in restoring health to all parts of the body.

Feel the stretch created in the muscles from your forearms all the way to the tips of your fingers as your arms reach the highest point. This part of the exercise opens qi flow in your small intestine, large intestine, and triple warmer meridians. As your hands drop downward, feel the stretch on the underside of your forearm. This movement opens the flow of qi in your lung, pericardium, and heart meridians.

The traditional Chinese concept of organs differs greatly from the Western idea of organs, which built its knowledge from dissection. Traditional Chinese medicine is much less concerned with the physical structure of an organ than with its observed function in the body. It is said, for example, that the pericardium, the casing around the heart, masters the vital circulation relating to the blood. Because of its function, the pericardium is considered one with the heart.

The triple warmer, to cite another example, doesn't even have a physical structure. The function of the triple warmer is to assist other organs. Keeping all passages open, it is a three-part "organ" that ensures that wastes are released from the body. Its upper burner, comprising the lungs and heart, disperses qi to the skin and muscles, supporting the immune system. Its middle burner, composed of the stomach and spleen, transports and transforms food and makes sure qi flows in the proper direction. Its lower burner, which includes the liver, gallbladder, kidneys, bladder, and intestines, transforms, transports, and releases fluids and waste products. It controls the downward movement of the intestines. The triple warmer is also the meridian through which *jing,* qi, and *shen* (the Three Treasures) are moved throughout the body.

In addition to stimulating the meridians of the organs mentioned above, Brushing Wind stimulates Conception Vessel 22 (see illustration on page 158) located in the depression between the clavicle bones. This point cools the throat and clears the voice, and is considered a gateway between the lower, middle, and upper *dantians*. When qi is flowing healthily through this area, a woman can speak her mind, express her feelings, and find her voice. Brushing Wind will help you to feel more integrated and connected to yourself.

The brisk swinging motion releases blockages within all of the meridians mentioned above, giving you an all-over healthy feeling. Get a great momentum going in this swinging action. It's so easy and feels so freeing that you may just want to do it forever.

Phoenix Eats Its Ashes

When and *if* you are able to touch your chin to your toes here, it is said that you will feel reborn, like the mythical bird, the Phoenix, rising from its ashes. The feeling of rebirth has been attributed to the exercise's powerful circulation of qi between the governing and conception vessels, major meridians that begin at the perineum, run along the center of our back and front respectively, and meet at the mouth. These two vessels are extremely important in Chinese medicine because they control the yin and yang of the entire body.

The governing vessel is known as the Sea of Yang because it regulates yang in the body. It controls the animation of the whole body and creates a connection between the heart and brain. The conception vessel regulates yin and is responsible for the proper flow of essence, blood, and fluid to nourish our life as well as that of a fetus.

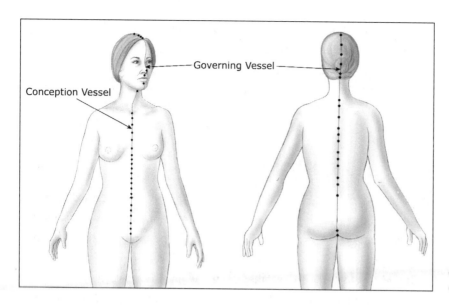

● *Conception and Governing Vessels*

Phoenix Eats Its Ashes also promotes functioning of the urinary bladder meridian, the longest in the body, which connects blood, bones, and all of our the internal organs.

Tigress Crouches Down

No matter what your age, feeling good about yourself is key to staying young. A woman can be twenty and still feel bad emotionally and physically. This exercise helps us stay "up" in so many ways, no matter how old we are. It stimulates Hundred Meeting point, the special energy center on the crown of the head that functions to "hold things up." Combined with the perineum point, it is used to treat dropped organs and hemorrhoids, and for raising the general energy levels of the body. When energy is flowing properly from the perineum point at your base up to the Hundred Meeting point, your life's purpose is clearer and you have an incredible feeling of autonomy.

Hundred Meeting point is stimulated frequently in the practice of qigong and is the gateway between the human body and the heavens. It has to do with being willing to live your life with purpose, to accept your lot in life and live it out with gusto. You can stimulate the Hundred Meeting point through self-acupressure as well. It keeps you "up" in a peaceful, youth-sustaining way. This exercise provides a tremendous rush of energy throughout your entire body

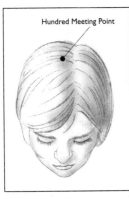

● *Hundred Meeting Point*

that can make you feel both grounded and as light as a feather. Forget caffeine, this exercise energizes you *and* helps you sleep at night!

By this stage of the warm-up, your qi is awake and your meridians are clear and flowing. All of your organs have been stimulated. You feel connected from the top of your head to your base, ready to move forward.

SET 1: TAPPING FOR QI

Massage is one of the most common practices in Chinese medicine and qigong. All three of the qigong exercises in this set achieve their benefits through gentle yet vigorous tapping of the body, a form of massage that further invigorates the flow of qi and blood through your meridians.

Blood is said to be the mother of qi, giving it nourishment, and qi the commander of blood, telling it where and how to move throughout the body. Without blood, qi has no substance and vice versa. According to Chinese medicine, blood is one of the most important components of a woman's health. Being more yin and having a tendency to be cold, women are naturally blood deficient. Added to that, once a month, women lose blood during menstruation. In Chinese medical thinking, blood circulates continuously, thus maintaining meridians and moistening our organs. It is thus essential to our health as women that we build the strength of our blood along with our qi. Set 1 and those that follow do just this.

Other benefits of tapping include stimulation of the lymphatic system, improved immunity, better elimination of waste, optimal respiration, boosted metabolism, and more.

One of several Chinese massage techniques is *tui na,* or "push pull," a tapping method that is simple and easy to perform. Highly effective for stimulating and strengthening many aspects of the body, it can be practiced anywhere, anytime. Through tapping, you direct qi where you want it to go, especially along meridians. Meridians can be separated into two main groups:

■ Yin meridians—Located on the inner arms and legs or the front of the torso, yin meridians govern the solid organs, which store energy, blood, and other substances, and are responsible for the essential functioning of the body. These include the spleen, kidneys, heart, pericardium, liver, and lungs.

- Yang meridians—Located on the outer arms and legs or the back and sides of the torso, the organs associated with the yang meridians are the hollow organs that disperse substances throughout the body. These include the meridians of the stomach, bladder, small intestines, triple warmer, gallbladder, and large intestines.

According to yin-yang theory, nature strives to harmonize opposites so that all may become balanced. As we are part of nature, humans need to maintain balance, too. Yin and yang are opposite qualities, so all of the so-called yang organs (which actively disperse) are said to have yin counterparts (which passively contain) and vice versa.

Traditional theory refers to these organs as husband and wife, reflecting their opposite but intricately entwined natures. Because this is a book for women and perhaps because I come from a family of five sisters, all of us very different, I refer to these counterparts as "sister organs." Sister organs are closely related and send energy back and forth to each other. Even though they are different, what happens to one affects the other.

Stimulated by tapping, the yin and yang meridians respond by moving stagnant qi from organs, circulating blood, and regulating qi more effectively. This form of self-massage is so powerful because it moves both qi and blood, which resolves existing aches and pains and also restores the body back to balanced good health.

Rag Doll Twist

The Rag Doll Twist opens up a tremendous energy flow and releases blockages of qi and blood. It invigorates your entire body and perks you up emotionally.

When you pat the area over your kidneys you stimulate the kidneys' sister organ, the bladder, as well as the adrenal glands on top of each kidney. When you pat your spleen you stimulate its sister organ, the stomach, and the nearby pancreas. You also stimulate the qi flow of the liver and its neighboring and sister organ, the gallbladder.

Have fun as you flop your hands and arms from side to side. As your momentum builds, you release more and more tension from the body and qi flows more freely up your spine.

- Rather than tapping the sides of your front and back, aim gently closed fists at two new spots. When your left fist hits the front of your body, make contact with your *dantian*. At the same time, your right fist hits the Life Gate Fire point, *mingmen*, connected to the health of your kidneys.

- As you turn at your waist, loosely swinging your arms, allow one fist to hit the top of your shoulder on a place midway between your neck and the tip of your shoulder. The other fist simultaneously hits *mingmen*, on your back. This variation helps release tension held in the shoulders, removing all "shoulds" from your "should-ers."

Thump Pump

This exercise is a wake-up call for your entire system. It affects your emotional as well as physical health, providing you with a heightened awareness and intolerance of unhealthy influences that come at you from all sides. Whether these influences are people, foods, or situations, Thump Pump helps you to reject those forces that undermine your well-being and to accept those that do.

As you thump, you prevent qi from stagnating in one part of the body by directing it to the *dantian* to be recycled. Increasing circulation of qi in the meridians brings vitality to your major organs. As you thump, move in the same direction that qi flows within the meridian. To ensure that you do this, follow the specified direction of thumping when doing these exercises.

Thumping up the outside of the arm stimulates the qi flow of the large intestine, small intestine, and triple warmer meridians, and:

resolves problems on the face

soothes neck pain

relieves toothache

promotes metabolism of water

disperses excess heat

balances body temperature

helps bowel elimination

Thumping down the inside of the arm stimulates the flow of qi within the lungs, heart, and pericardium meridians, and:

nurtures the spirit
clears the mind
creates calmness
nourishes the skin
promotes blood flow
creates gynecological wellness
strengthens and opens breathing capacity

Thumping on the muscles between your neck and the tip of your shoulder stimulates points on the gallbladder, large intestine, small intestine, and triple warmer meridians, and:

relieves neck tension
helps you make better decisions
balances body temperature
promotes metabolism of water

Thumping upward from the inside of your ankle stimulates the flow of qi within the meridians of the liver, spleen, and kidneys, and:

creates gynecological health
increases qi and blood flow
sparks the energy of all organ systems
optimizes digestive function
nourishes the ears, mouth, lips, and eyes
strengthens bones, muscles, and tendons

The next part of Thump Pump not only opens flow of qi within the meridians that cross the tapped areas but also opens the flow of lymph in these areas. Lymph, a clear fluid that contains wastes and proteins, comes from the interstitial fluid surrounding cells. It removes waste and brings your cells nourishment. Lymphatic fluid can only flow throughout your body with the aid of movement and massage. It helps maintain a strong immunity and healthy balance of other fluids in your body.

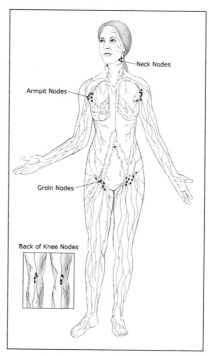

● *Lymphatic System*

To stimulate your lymphatic system and fight illness, pay special attention to the backs of the knees, groin region, armpits, and neck.

Beating the Heavenly Drum

Though there are many benefits of this simple exercise, including relieving headaches and preventing hair loss, one of the most immediate is to strengthen brain function, increasing memory and sharpening mental focus. With the newfound heightened awareness it brings, this movement indirectly helps you to trust more deeply in yourself and trust your intuition regarding others.

VARIATION ‖ Use your fingers to tap your entire scalp and face as well as the area at the base of your head called the Jade Pillow (see Back of Head Acupoints illustration page 159). This awakens your body, mind, and spirit, stimulating a multitude of acupoints located along the gallbladder, stomach, bladder, triple warmer, small intestine, large intestine meridians, and governing and conception vessels.

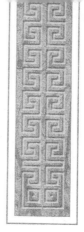

Vital Organs

IN SET 2, you harness the qi that is now flowing freely, directing it in a more focused way to your vital organs. This new flow to your organs provides increased health and energy.

SET 2: FIVE HEALING SOUNDS

The Five Healing Sounds integrate specific sounds with particular postures or movements. The purpose of combining sound with these postures and movements is to purify the qi of the organs and expel toxins. This set restores health and balance through vocalization of sounds, visualization of color, positive affirmations, and particular movements that stimulate organ function.

The Chinese system of healing through sound associates the sound with a particular emotion and position of the body. Sometimes you will experience one negative emotion more frequently than others, signifying that your organ is in some way unhealthy or out of balance.

Traditionally, the sound associated with each organ is believed to stimulate acupoints, which in turn influence the flow of qi within the internal organ's meridian. The healing sounds are widely used in China and have excellent clinical effects. Western research on how sound affects us physically is beginning to confirm the ancient linkage between sound and well-being.

The five sounds are done for five yin organs (heart, spleen, lungs, kidneys, and liver), but they also treat their five yang organ "sisters" (small intestines, stomach, large intestines, bladder, and gallbladder), with which they have a symbiotic relationship.

As mentioned above, the main functions of the yin organs are to create and store the essential substances of the body, which include qi, essence, blood, and fluids from the body.

The yin organ functions will be explained in greater depth. The functions of the yang organs are explained in the following chart:

Yang Organs	Organ Functions
Triple Warmer	has a name but no shape, regulates the functioning of all organs that govern water
Stomach	receives and ripens ingested foods and fluid
Small Intestine	separates the clear from the turbid, continues the process of separation of food that the stomach began
Large Intestine	moves the turbid (unuseful) parts of the food downward and absorbs water from the waste material
Urinary Bladder	receives and excretes water
Gallbladder	stores and secretes bile, rules decisions

● *Yang Organ Functions*

For many of us, especially Westerners, it may at first feel strange to make such "exotic" sounds. How was it ever determined, we may well wonder, that a particular sound benefits a particular organ?

While Western medicine studies what happens in the body mainly through external observation, such as dissection, traditional Chinese medicine also relies on internal observation—what people feel and say they feel, especially in relation to certain changes in the natural world. How do our bodies feel when it rains? When it is humid? At certain altitudes? In certain seasons and times of day? Our qi is intricately connected with the energy of nature.

One of the outward signs of internal experience is the expression of sounds. Humans have always made sounds when sick or experiencing stress, grief, or anger. These sounds relieve pressure on different organs, improving qi circulation in the meridians associated with the organs as well. Long ago, it was almost universally observed that when people were cold they tried to get warm by keeping their arms and legs close to their bodies, breathing deeply, and making certain sounds, in particular one similar to the kidney sound *"cherwee."* Not coincidentally, the function of the kidneys, according to Chinese medicine, is to warm and spark the energy of the body. Historical accounts also show that people have always emitted a *"shu"* sound, which is the liver sound, likened to blowing air on a cut to help stop bleeding and pain. Again, this makes sense, because a function of the liver is to govern the flow of blood, remove blockages, and thus release pain, promoting healing of a wound.

By trial and error, practitioners of Chinese medicine learned to focus these sounds we all made naturally, stimulating the innate healing capabilities of the body.

To understand how the healing sounds work, it is important to remember that we are all part of nature. Our bodies are made up of an interplay of five elements: wood, fire, earth, metal, and water. The five-element theory ascribes different sounds, emotions, colors, and qualities to the particular internal organs stimulated within this qigong set.

The illustration of the five elements and their associated organs shows solid arrows that signify the Nourishing (*shen*) Cycle. In this cycle, one organ creates and nourishes another. Broken lines, drawn in a star pattern between the elements, represent the Controlling (*ko*) Cycle whereby one organ controls the other.

Traditionally, an organ of the Nourishing (*shen*)

● *Five Element Diagram*

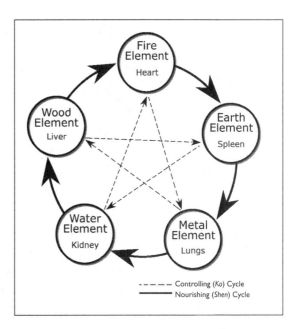

Cycle is considered a "mother" organ that nourishes its "child" organ, and an organ of the Controlling (*ko*) Cycle is considered a "grandparent" organ that controls its "grandchild" organ. In this text, I refer instead to the "grandparent" organ as the "father" because most Westerners think of the father as having the controlling role in the family.

The function of each organ is related to the proper functioning of all other organs. Vibrant health comes from a free and balanced flow of energy throughout all of your organs. These interrelationships represent a basic tenet of Chinese medical theory—all symptoms in the body are related, all organs affect other organs, and all of us contain elements of nature that must be balanced. The following list illustrates the basic relationships between the organs based on both cycles. Understanding the relationship between the elements helps us gain deeper insight into the inner workings of our bodies.

- Liver is governed by wood, nourished by water, controlled by metal.
- Heart is governed by fire, nourished by wood, controlled by water.
- Spleen is governed by earth, nourished by fire, controlled by wood.
- Lungs are governed by metal, nourished by earth, controlled by fire.
- Kidneys are governed by water, nourished by metal, controlled by earth.

Chinese medical theory teaches that excessive emotions can cause the organ qi to become blocked or deficient, in turn causing an imbalance within the organ's meridians. When the emotion becomes a chronic pattern in a person's life, illness is more likely. The pattern can also lead to weakened immunity, eventually blocking proper qi flow.

It's essential to remember that illness happens on an energetic or emotional level prior to manifesting physically. This underscores the preventive potential of qigong, which is believed to release, soothe, and remove energetic blockages or deficiencies before they have a chance to manifest on a physical plane.

It's not that it's bad to have certain emotions. Quite the contrary is true. All emotions need to be experienced and expressed. It's just that when we experience certain emotions excessively over a long period of time, physical problems arise within the associated organs. The Five Healing Sounds not only balance the level of emotion you feel but also transform negative emotions into positive ones. A balanced emotional state is of utmost importance and leads the body toward better health and longevity.

Creative visualization is an important aspect of the Five Healing Sounds set and is used to maximize the healing power of each exercise. Visualization has an actual physical effect on neuropeptides, chemicals that relay thoughts and emotions from the brain to the body, and vice versa. Neuropeptides directly affect the functioning of our organs and immune system. The immune system is affected by thoughts and actions of anger, sadness, worry, grief, and fear. Creative, positive visualizations improve qi flow, clear obstructions, and restore and maintain health.

VISUALIZATION TIPS ‖

- While working the qi of a particular organ, visualize yourself cleansing that organ. Bring good clean energy from the earth into the organ as you inhale, and remove any toxic energy as you exhale.
- Visualize a color attached to the breathing process. Simply "breathe in" the associated color of the particular organ:
    green for liver
    red for heart
    yellow for spleen
    white for lungs
    black or dark blue for kidneys
- Visualize any negative energy leaving the organ as you exhale.
- Make the sound and visualize directing it to the organ. Consult the diagram of the internal organs below so you know exactly where to concentrate your positive thoughts. This will help your sound find its mark!

Sound creates vibration and vibration influences the health of cells. Each sound and method of making the sound creates a particular vibration or a natural frequency that stimulates the specific organ. Be creative and have fun with your visualizations. Never underestimate the power of your mind.

As you practice, note the connection between the organ you are stimulating, the sensory organ it nourishes, and the tissue it controls according to the five elements.

- Liver nourishes eyes and tendons.
- Heart nourishes tongue and blood vessels.
- Spleen nourishes mouth and muscles.
- Lungs nourish nose, skin, and hair.
- Kidneys nourish ears, hair on head, and bones.

Using the Healing Sounds to Target an Unhealthy Organ

An organ's patterns of disharmony are caused not only from excessive negative emotion related to that organ but also from overworking, mental strain, and stress. If one of your organs is not functioning properly or needs special attention, choose the sound for that organ to help heal it. Repeat the sound up to thirty-six times. You may add as few or as many visualizations as you like to enhance the healing process of your vital organ. Also, don't be attached to saying the sound in a particular way. Allow your intuition to guide you. This is the independent, creative qigong spirit at work.

Additionally, you may choose to face the direction related to the particular organ according to the five-element theory. Face east for the liver, south for the heart, west for the lungs, and north for the kidneys. Use a consistent center in your practice space to the aid the spleen.

As you practice the whole workout, you may also choose to face north or west to strengthen yin energy, or face south or east to strengthen yang energy. Many qigong practitioners face east to promote personal growth because this direction relates to the wood element, which signifies growth. The best guidance I can give you is to experience each direction for yourself, notice any differences in how you feel when facing the different directions, and then choose the one that feels best to you.

The Liver Sound: Creates Free Flow of Energy and Blood

Located on your right side just below your diaphragm, the liver is one of the largest and most important organs in your body. Western medicine

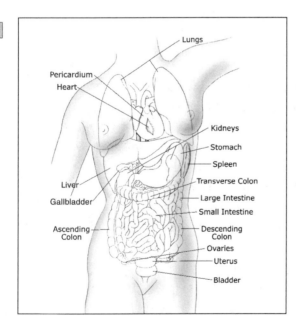

Lungs

Pericardium
Heart

Kidneys

Stomach

Spleen

Liver

Transverse Colon

Gallbladder

Large Intestine

Small Intestine

Ascending
Colon

Descending
Colon

Ovaries

Uterus

Bladder

recognizes the liver's role in detoxification and in cleansing the blood. Remarkably, the liver can physically regenerate itself.

In Chinese medicine, the liver rules the free flow and spread of qi and bodily substances. The liver controls bile secretion, harmonizes the emotions, moves and stores the blood, rules the tendons, shows itself in the nails, and is associated with the eyes. It is the sister organ to the gallbladder.

The liver is associated with the negative emotion of anger. The liver is also associated with the negative qualities of hostility and frustration and the positive virtues of kindness, generosity, and forgiveness. It is said that liver problems lead to anger, and we shout to release negative energy blocking the liver. If you or someone you know is always yelling and shouting, it probably indicates a liver energy imbalance. Release negative emotions through the Healing Sound for Liver and create more potential to experience positive emotions.

Other symptoms of liver imbalance include a greenish/yellowish tone of the eyes or skin. Since the liver blood nourishes and moistens the skin, when it is deficient the skin can become dry and itchy. This happens frequently during menopause.

The liver is of great importance in the later years of women's lives. It influences gynecological health through its relationship with the uterus and blood. The liver provides most of the blood that is stored in the uterus. A disharmony of the liver energy can lead to "coldness" in the uterus, a common cause of fertility problems. The qi of the liver is also responsible for moving blood, so the amount of liver qi is directly related to the available amount of liver blood.

When there is imbalance of the liver energy, there may be several patterns of disharmony within the same person at the same time. This is more common for the liver than for other organs. In the cycles of the five elements, the liver, kidneys, and heart are closely connected. When there are imbalances of the liver, this in turns causes problems with the kidneys and heart, and vice versa.

I can't emphasize enough how important it is to keep the qi and blood of your liver flowing freely and abundantly to experience vibrant health in the thirty-five-plus years. With all of the essential bodily functions the liver influences, you can imagine what a devastating effect a malfunctioning liver can have on your body. Practicing your healing sound is a step in the right direction for rectifying and preventing liver imbalance.

The Heart Sound: Strengthens the Mind and Pacifies the Spirit

The heart pumps blood throughout our bodies. Chinese medicine holds that the heart governs the blood vessels, houses the mind, stores the spirit, and opens into the tongue. The heart is like a relay system sending messages between all organ systems of the body. Its sister organs are the small intestine, triple warmer, and pericardium.

Many things can go wrong when the heart is out of balance, from gynecological problems to mental ones. The heart has a direct effect on the gynecological system because of its relationship with the blood and its flow. In practical terms, this means that the heart has to do with the quality and quantity of our blood, which governs our menstruation or lack thereof. The uterus is connected with the heart, which brings it blood and energy and also affects menstruation.

The heart houses the mind. How lucid and clear our mind is influences our emotional state as well. This helps to explain why emotions are such an important part of our experience during menstruation, pregnancy, childbirth, and menopause. For example, when there is a deficiency of blood in the uterus (after childbirth or in menopause), depression may ensue. Thus, for women experiencing symptoms caused by blood deficiency, it is essential to nourish heart blood.

The heart influences our spirit, how deeply we connect with our higher purpose and develop spiritually. It governs our communication skills, how we talk and what we talk about. The emotions most strongly affecting the heart are joy and sadness. The heart is also associated with the negative qualities of arrogance, cruelty, and hate, and the positive virtues of love and kindness. Excessive joy or laughter are believed to injure the heart because the body becomes overexcited. Laughing too much can lead to an increase of pressure on the heart. Pensiveness and worry agitate the heart and cause heart qi to "rebel" upward. This can result in scanty periods or infertility.

The Spleen Sound: Create a Vital Source of Life

The spleen is located on the upper left side of the torso just below the stomach. According to Chinese medicine, the spleen governs transformation and transportation of food and rules the muscles and flesh. The spleen opens into the mouth and is the sister organ to the stomach.

The spleen is associated with the negative emotions of overthinking. The spleen is also associated with worry, excess sympathy, pity, and anxiety, and, on the positive side, the virtues of fairness, compassion, and openness. We assist the functioning of our spleen through singing.

No matter what kind of food you ingest, if your spleen energy is disrupted, you will have difficulty absorbing nutrients from your foods. The spleen is the source of qi and blood and therefore is considered "the source of life."

The spleen makes the blood that is then transformed into female menstrual blood and averts painful periods. The spleen also holds blood in its place and so prevents symptoms such as excessive bruising. It holds other organs up and in place. A deficiency of spleen qi can lead to prolapse of the uterus or bladder.

Imbalances in the spleen lead to excess dampness, another big concern for women. When we have excessive dampness in our systems, we retain water and weight. Problems with the spleen can lead to excessive worry and you may either lose your appetite or eat too much as a result. You may find yourself talking a lot to others because talking releases negative energy and balances the spleen.

The Lung Sound: Nourish Your Breath

The lungs transmit oxygen to our bloodstream. According to Chinese medicine, lung energy rules the qi, moves and adjusts the water channels, rules the exterior of the body such as the skin, is reflected in the health of body hair, and is said to open to the nose. The lungs are the sister organ to the large intestines.

Lungs are predominantly associated with grief and also with the negative qualities of sadness and depression and the positive virtues of courage and righteousness. Unexpressed grief creates problems for the lungs. Excessive grief depletes you and may lead to stagnation of lung qi in the chest, indirectly affecting the breasts. Express your grief but don't wallow in it.

When someone cries too easily it indicates a lung energy imbalance. But crying actually helps reduce the negative energy and tension from the lungs. When we cry, our nose runs and fluids are created in the mouth. This gets rid of sadness in the lungs. The act of coughing is similar in that it also relieves tension from the lungs, especially during a cold or flu. Imbalance of the lung energy also has an indirect effect on blood, which is related to menstruation. When the qi governed by the lungs is depleted, it can lead to a dropped uterus, or if we experience too much grief and sadness, our menstrual flow stops.

The lung sound calms the body down during times of nervousness and opens the chest to ease breathing.

The Kidney Sound: Spark Your Life Gate Fire

Located on the back of the abdominal cavity, one on either side of the spine, the kidneys excrete urine and help regulate the content of water and blood in the body. They are considered the "root of life." They provide the foundation for the movement and transformation of water in the body, rule birth, development, and maturation, govern bones, and aid in the grasping of qi during inhalation. The health of the kidneys is reflected in the hair on the head and the health of the ears. The bladder is the kidneys' sister organ.

The kidneys are associated with the negative emotion of fear, which is related to the activity of the adrenal glands located just above them. They also relate to the positive virtues of gentleness and kindness.

The kidneys are usually the first organs in our bodies to feel the effects of stess. Extreme levels of stress over an extended period of time can have disastrous affects on the kidneys, producing a fight-or-flight syndrome that catapults you into a constant heightened state of alert. Without the existence of potential danger, this state makes no sense, makes you uncomfortable in your own skin, and causes damage to the functioning of the kidneys and the immune system.

The fight-or-flight sensation—heart pumping, knots in your stomach, adrenaline rushing to the legs—is a classic example of the typical anxiety-driven, stress-induced condition in which many women find themselves. You may never have experienced such extreme reactions. Nonetheless, symptoms of chronic stress, though less severe, are no less damaging. Over time, stress takes its toll on your kidneys.

Qigong practice releases us, calming us and promoting the proper functioning of the parasympathetic nervous system to bring us into a normal, balanced, and centered state.

The kidneys have a direct effect on the gynecological system. The kidneys provide the uterus with essence, the material basis of menstrual blood, which the Chinese call period water. The kidneys, through the adrenal glands, are a source of both water and fire. The kidneys also play an important role in the production of vital hormones such as adrenaline, aldosterone, cortisol, and natural steroids.

Kidney deficiency is at the root of many women's health problems. Deficiency in the kidneys can deplete both water and fire, which influences the uterus in its storage of blood. This condition often combines with blood deficiency to create a host of symptoms. This is commonly the situation for a woman during menopausal years.

A basic precept of Chinese medicine is that the kidney essence (*jing*) decreases as we get older. Consequently, women need to strengthen kidney essence during perimenopause (the time before our periods cease), menopause, and postmenopause. Qigong practice naturally strengthens and balances both the yin and yang aspects of the kidneys and thus the uterus, which is located in the area of a woman's lower *dantian*.

Rebalancing of kidney energy results in:

a strong back
vibrant and plentiful energy
feeling sexier
warm hands and feet
greater sense of security
clear and focused thoughts
better hearing
being fearless and forthright
healthy hair

Kidney Rub for Life

The kidney energy is precious to the Chinese. It is believed that when kidney qi is gone, so is life. Chinese medicine provides many exercises, herbs, and treatments to nourish and protect kidney qi. It is my belief that high stress levels in our society and a lack of practices to protect our kidney energy are the cause of increased kidney disease. Because the kidneys do not regenerate, any disease or damage to the kidneys is permanent. For this reason, it is essential to keep your kidneys in the best shape possible.

Do a daily kidney rub to stimulate the health of your kidneys. This is especially good during the winter months when your kidneys need as much warmth as possible or during times of extreme fear or insecurity. The exercise awakens the *jing* energy, the essential life energy stored in the kidneys, and the vitally important *mingmen* point located between the two. The Kidney Rub for Life also stimulates the urinary bladder meridian, which balances the yin and yang of the kidneys. Treatment of this meridian alleviates urinary problems, low back pain, and excess heat conditions such as bladder infections.

How to Do the Kidney Rub for Life

With loosely closed fists, rub the back of your hands over your lower back until the area feels warm, even hot. At the same time, visualize qi circulating

● *Kidney Rub for Life*

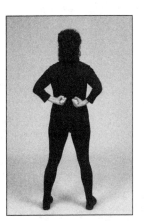
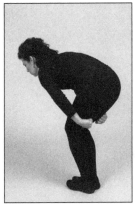
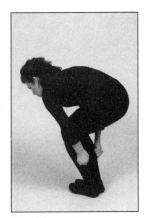
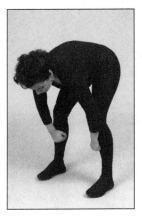
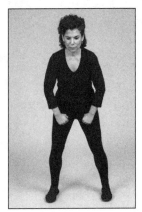

Qigong for Staying Young

in your kidneys. Continue rubbing down the center and backs of both legs, over the sides of your legs, then over the tops of your feet, up the insides of your legs, over your hips and to your lower back once again. Do this over and over for approximately three minutes per day for however many days per week you are inclined.

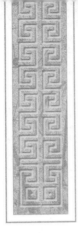

Cultivating Qi

IN PREVIOUS SETS, you woke up your body's qi and began to feel its flow throughout the meridians, using it to purify your vital organs. Now you are ready to refine your experience of qi. Cultivating its flow, you become even more aware of its healing action in your body.

SET 3: PLAYING WITH QI

In this set you are learning to discover, cultivate, circulate, and conserve your qi. As you do these exercises, look for movement within the calmness and calmness within the movement. What does this mean? In qigong, so much is happening even when nothing appears to be happening. Even when you're not moving, your qi is flowing.

In today's busy world, we are barraged with noise, chatter, and endless amounts of sensory information. As we go about our daily lives, many of us have a hard time just being silent and standing still. When we stop running, both literally and figuratively, and observe our qi, we discover an inner peace. We discover ourselves.

Being anxious or stressed causes shallow breathing, which deprives our body of the qi it needs to operate at full capacity. As you do the exercises in this set, take gentle, deep, and slow breaths into your lower abdomen. Take long, smooth inhalations and exhalations. Breathe naturally and without force. Breathing this way balances and harmonizes your qi.

As you play with the qi in this set, move your hands slowly into the position, coordinate your breathing with your movements, and allow your movements to come from your *dantian*. This creates a smooth flow of qi and blood throughout the body, calms the heart and mind, and promotes overall relaxation. It also ensures that you don't move ahead of your qi. This is an important rule to remember when doing any of the slower-paced qigong exercises.

Besides breathing shallowly, a common mistake beginners make while Playing with Qi is to move their arms and hands totally separately from their torsos and the rest of their bodies. There is also a tendency to move one's body in a rigid and mechanical way. The following suggestions will help you avoid these pitfalls.

Helpful Hints

For qi to really flow, move your arms in a soft, relaxed manner. Let your arms be slightly rounded as they move out from your shoulder. This roundness extends out into your relaxed, slightly open fingertips.

To be sure you are "moving as one," hold one arm out in front of your heart, keeping it rounded with your palm facing toward you. Relax your arm in this position, but don't move it. Now place one foot in front of the other with your weight on your back leg. Slowly shift your weight from back to front. Without altering the distance between your arm and your heart and without moving your shoulder joint, move the arm in a counterclockwise circle. Achieve this simply by shifting your weight from your back foot to your front foot and allowing the movement to emanate from your *dantian*. Next, attempt this in a clockwise direction. When this feels easy, switch feet and arms and repeat. You will be amazed at how much you can move your arm in a circular fashion without ever moving your arm from your shoulder joint.

Feeling Qi

This exercise shows you how all qigong movements feel when they emanate from your waist, or *dantian*. When you move from your *dantian*, you promote free circulation throughout your entire body, strengthen your qi and blood, calm your heart and spirit, and take a giant step toward cultivating your qi in a powerful new way. The more you feel the qi, the more your qi is moving, and the more you relax.

With this exercise, qi moves from one hand to the other. Many experience the sensation as a push and pull between magnets. When you pull your hands apart, you feel a force holding your palms together. When you push your hands together, you feel a certain resistance. This sensation comes from the interaction of the qi that is flowing out of the acupoints on each of your hands. Heavy, tingling, and warm, this is referred to as thick qi.

Thick qi is precisely the energy you apply to yourself to create healing within your body. Feeling the qi allows you to focus your qi where you want it to go. You may imagine you are pulling taffy between your hands while doing this exercise. Whatever image you use, visualize the qi you generate to enhance your sense of its presence.

Different exercises provide varying levels of the "thick qi" sensation. You may experience a "sticky" sensation between each hand. The variations depend on the particular area of the body where vital energy is flowing, combined with your ability to relax and allow it to flow freely. Sometimes you'll feel many sensations and sometimes none at all. Be patient, practice every day, and your energy will develop in its own time. Even if you don't experience any of the sensations described above, qi may still be flowing.

As you progress through the exercises, you may begin to feel as if you were larger than you actually are. This is because you are extremely relaxed, blood is flowing freely, and your qi is circulating in and out through all of your acupoints. If you begin to feel smaller, this is good, too, and is due to the concentration of qi in your *dantian*.

All of the following sensations indicate you are "realizing your qi":

heat in your palms
tingling, aching, or itchiness in your fingers

numbness

swelling or soreness in your hands

the sensation of a passing breeze

a magnetic pull between your hands

a thick or heavy feeling in your hands.

If you feel unpleasant cold spots in your body, this means you are carrying too much tension and negativity. However, if feel you pleasantly cool it means that qi is circulating well.

Feeling the Three Seas

VARIATION ‖ As you do your Feeling Qi exercise, see if you can feel the energy fields extending out from all three of your *dantians* rather than just from the lower *dantian*. Do this by shifting your hands from in front of your lower abdomen, the Sea of Energy, to the center of your chest, the Sea of Tranquility, to in front of your forehead, the Sea of Spirit. Breathe in as your hands move outward and breathe out as your hands move toward each other. As your hands move in and out in front of these three areas, sense the variations in energetic sensations at each *dantian* field.

Most people can feel qi, but more people than you would think can actually *see* it. Stay open to whatever your particular experience might be. Seeing is believing, and qi might appear as a translucent ray of light extending from your fingers, a white haze flowing around you, white cloudy energy in your field of vision, crystallized forms in the air, or a glimpse of light within the shadows of your hands. Don't be alarmed if "a light goes on" during your practice! Whatever you see, even if you see nothing, it is all right.

Fluffing White Clouds

As you do this exercise, you may experience your qi as a gentle fire burning in your *dantian*. This tells you that qi is flowing vigorously. You may also feel an increasing tingling, itching, or sensitivity in your hands. This means qi is flowing freely and stagnant qi is being released.

VISUALIZATION TO RELEASE STAGNANT QI ‖ Breathe naturally and imagine you are moving the qi up and down in front of you, promoting qi flow all around you. Next, as you inhale, bring your hands upward and visualize yourself drawing qi from the earth into the center of your palms. See the qi circulating throughout and penetrating your entire being. When you exhale and bring your hands toward the earth, see harmful, stagnant qi breaking loose and send it down into the ground. You may want to say the following affirmation either aloud or silently, to yourself: My hands are filled with vibrant and vital energy. I am sending positive and powerful virtues deep within me on my inhalation. I am sending negativity into the earth on my exhalation. I am creating abundant qi within and around me, with each and every moment celebrating my wholeness.

Fluffing White Clouds stimulates the endocrine glands, structures that have a huge effect on the overall functioning of our systems. The endocrine system controls the timing of when you wake up, how much sexual desire you have, the amount of calcium in your body, your resistance to disease, the rate of your metabolism, how you age, and even, some scientists argue, your ability to have spiritual experiences. Endocrine glands are the masters of the body and when there is dysfunction in one of these glands it can upset the entire system. Strengthening the functioning of the endocrine glands is key to living a long and healthy life.

Swan Stretches Her Wings

Swan Stretches Her Wings allows you to connect with the energies of heaven and earth and at the same time harmonize the forces of yin and yang within your system. When your palm pushes up to the sky, yang qi enters. When it pushes to the earth, yin qi enters. As you swirl your arms across your middle *dantian,* you feel a magnetic pull between your hands and it is almost as if your whole body becomes a yin-yang symbol. When your hands hold the imaginary qi ball over your middle *dantian,* the qi of the earth and sky mix together with your human qi. This motion draws on the strength of planets in the solar system, as well as planet earth. Sun and earth also embody masculine and feminine qualities respectively, so through this movement you balance these qualities within yourself. No small task!

Any qigong movement like this one that stimulates energy in the center of the torso opens the flow of qi to the spleen and stomach and thus affects the aspects of you that relate to these organs. As you have already learned, the spleen and stomach are related to overthinking and obsessive behavior. They also govern the transportation and transformation of food in the body. When this area of the body is opened through qigong, you will feel more easygoing, better able to make quick decisions and to listen to your own needs. Literally and figuratively, you will feel yourself digesting things more easily.

Any qigong movement in which you stretch, twist, or bend also stimulates the torso. The torso opens the flow of qi to the liver and gallbladder meridians and their related organs. Since these organs have to do with anger and frustration, stretching the torso allows you to manage how much anger you feel toward others and how quickly you get frustrated and angry with yourself.

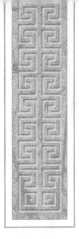

Mind Intent

IN QIGONG, mind intent is the mental focus we cultivate in order to direct our qi and manifest our goals. In this set, we begin to concentrate our mind's intent in order to create greater balance within. In the words of a qigong proverb, "Where the mind goes, the qi will follow."

SET 4: QI MIND, QI BODY

This set starts off with Woman Connects with Heaven and Earth to open the yin-yang connection between your body and the diametrically opposing forces of nature. After this, you will learn how to cultivate your heaven/earth connection and mind intent practice through the standing and walking Yi-Chuan exercises.

Woman Connects with Heaven and Earth

This exercise stimulates the upper spine and in so doing stimulates the nerves closest to the brain, affecting your emotions, mental state, and memory. The forward and backward bending of your spine stimulates the entire central axis of your body and benefits your kidneys and spleen as well. This in turn promotes happiness and tranquility, and the health of your back, neck, and hip regions.

The origin of the movement is in yin-yang theory as applied to three fundamental concepts in ancient Chinese philosophy: the three powers of nature—heaven, earth, and the human. All three of these powers affect and influence the other. True health exists when you adjust your own body according to the principles of yin and yang and get in sync with the yin and yang of heaven and earth. When there is an imbalance in the forces of heaven, tornados, hurricanes, and other natural disasters result. When imbalance occurs on the earth, we have earthquakes and rivers change direction. So, too, when there is imbalance in the human body, illness takes hold.

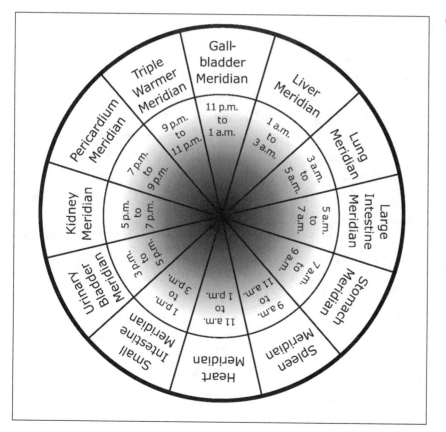

● *Chinese Body Clock*

Existing as we do between heaven and earth, humans receive energy from both sources. In this exercise, we draw energy from the earth upward from our Bubbling Well points out of a root spot slightly below our feet. We connect the positive and negative poles, transmitting the current that activates life. Daily, we use this energy to live. Over time and with practice, we can learn to store it and draw upon it in times of need.

Women are influenced by the powers of the sun and moon and the magnetic field of the earth. The circulation of qi in our body is affected by the forces of nature and by how we interact with these forces. A prime example of this is the connection of our menstrual cycle to the waxing and waning of the moon.

As you perform the movements of Woman Connects with Heaven and Earth, become increasingly aware of your connection to nature and the profound meaning behind your movements. Notice how these simple gestures have a deep effect on your health and balance in the life you create for yourself. Be aware, too, of how you feel as you practice in different seasons, and at different times of the day.

The Chinese medicine body clock is based on the belief that qi flows through our twelve different meridians with differing intensity in a twenty-four-hour period. Each meridian remains particularly active for a span of two hours. Refer to the clock to understand why you may feel a certain way during a particular time of the day. Use it, too, to choose what time of the day to practice based upon the particular organ that you would like to strengthen. One of the most common occurrences I've noticed in regards to the body clock is how night coughing seems always to occur between 3:00 and 5:00 A.M., which is the lung time. Furthermore, it is important to get to sleep by 11:00 P.M. to give your gallbladder and liver their proper rest. The body clock also explains why some artists do their best work in the wee hours of the morning, as the liver is connected with creativity. It is so common for people to get tired around 5:00 P.M. when kidney energy is weakest, and to need to evacuate their intestines by 7:00 A.M.

Consult the body clock to confirm or expand your experience.

Yi-Chuan Standing And Walking Exercises

The standing and walking exercises in this set are a type of qigong called Yi-Chuan (pronounced "ee- chwan"). Yi means "mind." Chuan means "fist." Thus, when you practice the exercises in this set, you are creating a kind of "mind fist," physical strength gained by honing the intention of your mind. Yi-Chuan teaches the practitioner how to respond naturally to whatever life might throw her way and to concentrate the spirit and stabilize the mind. By learning first to use the mind, the body becomes stronger, more whole and balanced. The exercises in this set are akin to meditations.

All of your qigong practice thus far has shown that true power comes from greater awareness, not outward appearance or strong muscles. Health, strength, and beauty come from within and from the yin and yang power of nature all around us.

The Yi-Chuan exercises help you maximize health, stimulate, develop, and bring forth your natural instinctive abilities, and deal with the challenges of daily life, extreme stress, aggression, or injury by maintaining your center.

Do you ever feel that the pressures of your daily existence have you running around like a chicken with its head cut off? The practice of Yi-Chuan fosters the ability to find an appropriate response to stress that is in harmony with yourself and your surroundings. Through Yi-Chuan practice, you can build a life in which action stems from inaction and stillness is the base of each movement. With practice of Yi-Chuan, when you act to face the challenges of life, you will do so from a turtle's place of deep calm and balance.

The exercises below help you integrate the mind with the body, develop qi, and focus intent. The purpose of each movement includes healing, self-defense, and spiritual awakening. When you are doing these exercises, don't push it. It is said that qi behaves like water; it can't be pushed, but it can be led. When you try to push qi, it floods into the wrong pathways. When qi is led it flows smoothly and without stagnation.

At this point in the workout, you have some understanding of what qi is, and of the quality of your own qi when you do your workout. As you perform Set 4, be aware of how strong your qi is and how smoothly it is flowing. The more communication you have between your yi and your qi, your mind and your energy, the better you will be able to manifest movements. When your yi is strong, your qi will be strong. How do you know when your mind is strong? The first sign is that you feel calm. This calmness means you are not easily distracted. You see things clearly and experience tremendous focus and concentration in your qigong practice and your life.

Standing Like a Tree

Standing meditation is an important foundation of qigong practice. Standing Like a Tree in particular is a powerful method of self-healing, activating qi to break down chronic blockages of energy. Standing practice develops more abundant qi, which you can send yourself through your hands to yourself for self-healing purposes. When you practice this exercise, you become stronger and healthier, forging a connection between the yin energy of the earth and the yang energy of the heavens.

Standing meditation develops a sensation of buoyancy, a fullness within the body that can be likened to a ball filled with air. In this exercise, you are filled with qi, creating a strong force evenly distributed across the surface of your body. Highly developed practitioners can use this force to repel objects and people without even touching them.

Even if you never achieve this "magical" ability, practicing the standing exercises will dramatically strengthen your force field. You may notice that people and situations that used to get under your skin no longer affect you in the same way. With this practice, your qi becomes thicker, protecting you from negative forces, even including germs that cause sickness.

This development of buoyant qi promotes health within the physical body and lessens the chance of injury. As we get older and become more prone to bone fracture, buoyant qi protects us. The buoyant qi, combined with the rooting developed from standing postures, reduces chances of falling. Standing Like a Tree also increases your sense of who is coming up behind you and can be helpful in protecting you from impending danger.

Make sure you feel healthy and fairly happy, not sick or angry as you begin these postures.

As you do your standing meditation, imagine that you are bringing energy from the heavens above down through your body and into the earth, promoting general well-being.

The qi in your body flows much as your blood flows through your arteries and veins. Move slowly from one position to the next so as not to get ahead of this flow. Experiment with moving quickly and then slowly so you can see the difference. Notice how your muscles become tense when you move too fast.

Be aware that standing meditation can stimulate the movement of your bowels. It's normal to need to empty your bowels or expel gas after doing the exercise. Be aware, too, that you may experience vibrating, shaking, or sudden jerking as you stand. This is a good thing. It means qi blockages are shaking loose. You may also feel heavy during your exhalation. This indicates that your qi is sinking down to the acupoints on the center of the soles of each foot, connecting you with the yin energy of the earth.

It's also common to begin to feel extraordinarily tall while you Stand Like a Tree. This means that you're relaxed, qi is circulating and flowing freely throughout your body, and is moving out from the crown of your head. The exercise promotes connection to the heavens, opening you to greater spiritual awareness that connects you with the yang energy from above.

Don't be surprised if you feel aching, pain, or numbness while doing your standing practice. This is a common experience. In fact, it indicates that your qi has been activated and a breakthrough of blockages is occurring.

Each of the eight Standing Like a Tree postures stimulates a different combination of acupoints, and so a different center of energy in your body. When your energy is flowing freely it creates a wall, or buffer, around you. This wall allows you to keep qi inside your body, preventing it from being lost.

VISUALIZATION ‖ Standing Like a Tree helps develop harmony between you and nature. The following visualization deepens this connection:

When you finish your standing meditation, stand comfortably with your eyes open, hands relaxed, back straight, mouth closed, and tongue resting gently on the roof of your mouth. Inhale and visualize energy being drawn up through the center of the bottoms of your feet from roots in the ground. See your spine as the trunk of the tree and continue this visualization by bringing the energy up from your feet, through your spine and up to the crown of your head. Upon exhalation, see the energy flowing down the front center of your body, out through the bottom center of each foot, down to the roots, and back into the earth. Repeat this three times and then stand with a quiet mind, noticing the sensations and feelings created. Feel how your spine creates a connection between the earth and the heavens and your arms are like branches reaching out for light to transform into energy. Feel the connection to the earth, the heavens, and to yourself, as you realize your intimate relationship to nature.

Walking Like a Turtle

While Standing Like a Tree is more of a yin exercise because there is little movement, Walking Like a Turtle is more of a yang exercise. This system of balanced, meditative walking is an essential counterpart to the standing meditation. Walking Like a Turtle is a way of circulating and conserving qi. As you walk forward and backward, you shift your weight from one foot to the other, from the front of your foot to the back, and move from side to side. All of these shifts stimulate and balance the flow of yin and yang. As you can see, even within a yang exercise yin exists, and vice versa. This is because yin and yang are relative and dynamic, never absolute or static.

The Chinese believe that the universe is made up of the opposite forces of yin and yang, which must balance each other. Yin and yang are polar opposites that exist within all of nature. If yin and yang fall out of balance, nature finds a way to create balance once more, sometimes resorting to extremes. Disaster and disease can occur if yin and yang remain extremely imbalanced for too long. On the other hand, great power and goodness occurs when yin and yang interact smoothly and harmoniously.

When yang energy is at a healthy level, there is warmth, vitality, healthy metabolism, and willpower. When yang is weak there is coldness, dampness, stagnation, low energy, and slow metabolism, and lack of motivation.

Women naturally have more yin in their systems, so it is usually the goal of qigong practice to bring us into a state of balance by nourishing our yang energy. When I say that women are naturally yin, this means that we are *usually* more introverted, soft, cold, blood deficient, dry, and internally focused than men. The goal of qigong practice for women is to balance those tendencies, to warm us up, strengthen our blood, help us to speak our minds, gently and fairly and at appropriate times. We often need to develop an outer shell when necessary for self-preservation and self-protection. A healthy yin-yang balance helps us come into our own, manifesting what we want, need, and deserve in our lives.

Walking Like a Turtle teaches you to balance the physical, emotional, and spiritual components of your yin and yang energies. As we walk, we balance the inside with the outside, deepening our relationship to nature. We balance our female aspects with those aspects of ourselves that are male, and our subconscious with the conscious aspects of our being. Yin and yang energy balances within our bodies as we shift the energy from one hand to the other, one side of the body to the other, and one foot to the other. This exercise helps us to go with the flow of what is happening in our lives.

Walking Like a Turtle can help you manifest your wants and desires. When something you want is in your mind—whether it be to find a new career, have a child, or build your dream house—it is in a yin state and can't yet be seen. With a concerted effort, you manifest what's in your mind and it comes into being, into physical form. It is then in a yang state. Manifestation from a state of yin to yang, nonexistence to existence, starts with the idea (yin) and moves into existence in a concrete form (yang). Both are needed for your intention to germinate and flower.

Physically, we must all balance the qualities of passive and active, softness and hardness, slowness with quickness. In the walking exercise, you shift the forces of yin and yang within yourself. When one foot has all of the weight on it, that foot is considered to be full, or yang. At the same time the other foot is empty, or yin. As you walk, your body balances the opposite forces within itself to reach a place of equilibrium. By doing this, you strengthen and balance your body and give it the necessary resources to ward off attacks from external factors such as viruses, cold, and heat, as well as attacks from within yourself that stem from negative emotions such as fear or anger.

In addition to balancing of the yin and yang energies of our body, Walking Like a Turtle develops a special resilience in the body that is considered to be a secret to the prevention of sports injuries. It is a way to infuse your whole body with qi—your organs, your meridians, right under your skin—providing you with protection against daily physical, emotional, and energetic stresses.

As your practice develops, your movements may feel slow and you may feel as if you're floating. Enjoy this sensation. It means your qi is flowing through your governing and conception vessels and reaching the Hundred Meeting point on the crown of your head.

VISUALIZATION || While most women do have more yin than yang, many have overdeveloped yang in response to the pressures of our modern lives. If you need to stop running and start feeling, this exercise will help. Some of us have created a hard wall around ourselves in response to the stress of the outside world. This hardness indicates there's too much yang in your system and it is time to soften, to fully breathe again. Turn dryness into moistness and hardness into softness as you bring springtime to your body. You may choose to say the following affirmation: *I feel myself opening to the beauty around me. I know when to trust and when to shy away. I am ready to experience the true joy and succulent sweetness of life.*

As you practice Walking Like a Turtle, imagine a seed within you begin to sprout, and bud, then to blossom into a beautiful flower. As the petals of the flower unfold, you open to the infinite possibilities that exist within. Allow your inner beauty and unique personality to express itself in all their splendor, for all the world to see.

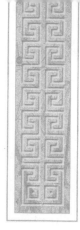

Hormone Power

THOUGH there is no exact equivalent in Chinese thought to the Western notion of hormones, Chinese medicine does have a notion of prenatal essence, or *jing*. Traditionally, Chinese medicine holds that prenatal essence can be converted into qi to stimulate the proper function of the physical body and promote overall vitality. *Jing* affects activity, thinking, growth, and metabolism and is directly related to the strength of your qi. For our purposes, *jing* can be equated with the hormones produced by our endocrine glands. Like *jing*, hormones determine longevity and whether a person is healthy or sick. Hormones have an effect on our emotions and mood and play a large part in whether we are depressed. Learning how to affect the production of your hormones through stimulation of the endocrine glands can produce positive results in all aspects of your being. This set helps you strengthen that essence.

SET 5: ENERGIZE ENDOCRINES

Set 5 stimulates endocrine gland function and helps you:

> adjust to the aging process
> mitigate hot flashes
> reduce high blood pressure
> strengthen bones
> develop mental clarity
> increase bladder control
> reduce vaginal dryness
> maintain an even keel emotionally

Hormones are complex chemical messengers secreted from the endocrine glands and transported by the blood and lymph. They have extremely powerful and profound effects on the function of the human body. According to Chinese medicine, both the kidney and the liver govern growth and reproduction and are thus considered intimately associated with the body's endocrine system. The kidneys do this by providing vital essence that nourishes the bones and enhances sexual growth. The liver does this through its role as a wood element which promotes growth and the circulation of blood thoughout the body.

When young it is important to balance your body's production of hormones. When you are older it is of utmost importance to increase their production because many of the glands' functions slow down with age. Qigong practice encourages your body to naturally balance hormones. During and after menopause, a boost in hormone levels, when properly directed, leads to increased qi production, nourishes the brain, and raises the vitality of your spirit.

Qigong masters believe that treatment of one of the endocrine glands treats them all, activating our full potential.

Hormones made in one gland send signals via body fluids to our organs and to other endocrine glands. While some glands do work on their own, many others are interdependent, engaging in complex interactions. These relatively small structures have a huge effect on overall health, to the point that the malfunctioning of one gland can throw everything off. The endocrine system includes the pituitary, hypothalamus, pineal, thyroid, parathyroid, thymus, adrenals, pancreas, and ovaries (testicles are also an endocrine gland).

Stimulate the glands in this set by sending them healing energy through your hands and love and attention via your mind intent. As you practice, visualize the gland in as much detail as you can and breathe deeply to heighten its qi. Most people notice subtle or profound differences in how they feel after practicing this exercise set. You may experience a tingling sensation after stimulating the endocrine glands, or otherwise sense that the energy of your glands has changed even though you have not touched them physically.

Pituitary, Hypothalamus, and Pineal Glands

The pituitary, called a master gland because it has a controlling influence over many of the other endocrine glands, is a small, gray, round structure about the size of a chickpea. It is attached to the base of the brain and is located at the level of the eyes. The pituitary secretes numerous hormones that regulate major processes of the body.

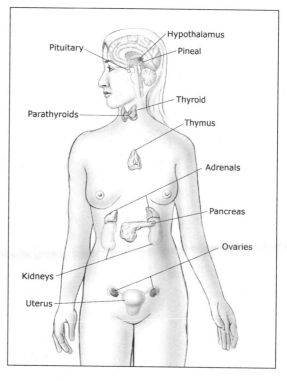

● *Endocrine Glands*

In Chinese medicine, the pituitary gland is associated with the *yintang* point (see illustration page 159) located between the eyebrows, also known as the third eye. This area relates to internal awareness and consciousness and its stimulation promotes the ability to see auras, the energy fields surrounding our bodies.

Together with the hypothalamus, the pituitary gland works to control many normal functions such as sleep, appetite, body temperature, sexual maturation, and reproduction.

Pituitary hormones greatly affect female physiology, influencing aspects such as growth, the health of sex organs, stimulation of eggs from the ovaries, contractions during childbirth, milk production during breast-feeding, fluid balance, blood pressure, salt retention, the protein of the certain bones, and the activity of the thyroid and adrenal glands.

The hypothalamus is located in the center of the brain, near the pituitary. Even though some sources don't consider it an endocrine gland, others do, and I have included the hypothalamus in this category because it shares many functions of a gland. In addition to the endocrine functions it governs with the pituitary, the hypothalamus helps to regulate your biological clock and sleeping patterns. There are a total of one hundred internal "clocks" located in almost every organ, tissue, and in many of the cells in your body, all synchronized by the hypothalamus. Secretions of the hypothalamus also help control water balance, sugar and fat metabolism, body temperature regulation, and secretion of other endocrine glands. The pituitary and the hypothalamus integrate sympathetic and parasympathetic activities of the nervous system, regulating the rhythms of the body that control when we wake and sleep, when we menstruate, and when we conceive.

Like the pituitary, the pineal gland has also been referred to in ancient cultures as the third eye and the heavenly eye. French philosopher René Descartes likened the pineal gland to the seat of the human soul, the location of what we call the mind. It is also thought to be related to the crown chakra (Hundred Meeting point), which relates to spiritual awareness and development of a higher consciousness. The pineal gland plays several significant roles in human functioning and only recently has the role of this tiny red pinecone-shaped gland become understood.

Located deep within the brain, the pineal secretes melatonin, a powerful body chemical believed to suppress electrical brain activity and regulate daily body rhythms, most notably the day/night cycle known as our circadian rhythm. It has been suggested that a balance of melatonin prevents jet lag and seasonal affective disorder. This hormone has a stimulatory effect on the immune system and may play a role in cancer prevention. In Chinese medicine, the pineal gland has long been thought to control acceleration of sexual growth and to slow the aging process. The activation of the pineal gland is critical to maintaining vibrant energy as well as a youthful and vital state of being.

As you emit healing qi to the pituitary, hypothalamus, and pineal glands in your brain, visualize for yourself a positive result of improved endocrine function.

Thyroid and Parathyroid Glands

The butterfly-shaped thyroid gland is at the base and front of the neck. Weighing almost one ounce, it consists of two lobes, one on each side of the windpipe. Every organ in your body, including the heart, lungs, stomach, and intestines, skin, hair, and nails, brain, and sexual organs, needs thyroid hormone to function. Together with the parathyroid, the thyroid regulates the body's metabolism and calcium balance. It promotes normal development from infancy through childhood and into our later years.

The thyroid influences basal metabolic rate and indirectly influences growth and nutrition. It is benefited by saliva in the mouth, which increases through practice of qigong. Saliva is called divine water in Chinese medicine and contains chemicals that help maintain vibrant health when swallowed. As saliva is formed during your workout, swallow it with the knowledge that it is benefiting overall health.

The parathyroid glands are four small oval-shaped endocrine glands, two lying behind each of the thyroid gland lobes in the neck. The parathyroid glands produce a hormone that helps to regulate calcium and phosphorus levels in your blood. Appropriate levels of calcium are essential to maintaining healthy muscles, bones, and nerves. Overproduction of parathyroid hormone leads to hyperparathyroidism, the symptoms of which are known as moans, groans, stones, and bones.

"Moans" are psychological symptoms such as irritability, depression and general mental disturbances. "Groans" are physical symptoms such as nausea or abdominal pain. "Stones" are formed in the urinary track from overproduction of calcium. "Bones" are symptoms of thin bones, bone pain, and fractures as a result of the parathyroid drawing more calcium out of the bones than is being replaced. This can be especially serious in aging women as the bones lose much of their calcium, becoming brittle and susceptible to fracture. Balancing parathyroid hormone levels increases strength of bones as you age.

When emitting qi to your thyroid and parathyroid, focus on symptoms you may have that are ruled by these glands and envision the glands' radiant health.

‖ Hold your neck erect but not stiff. Keep it centered without inclining to the left or the right. Slowly stretch your head forward and backward, then side to side. These movements increase the functioning of the thyroid and parathyroid glands. At the same time you do these movements, emit qi from your hands to these precious glands. Repeat three times in each direction.

Thymus Gland

A small gland located in the chest just under the upper part of your breastbone, the thymus extends upward into the root of the neck. This gland reaches its full size during puberty. As we age, the thymus gland naturally shrinks, becoming less effective.

The thymus is a critical component of the body's defense response to disease and is essential in the development and maturation of a specific type of white blood cell: the T-lymphocyte, commonly known as a T-cell. There are many forms of T-lymphocytes but their basic purpose is to fight off disease at the cellular level. The full importance of the thymus in adults is still not clear and it is likely that the thymus is undervalued by the medical and scientific world. For this reason, it is well worth our time to do what we can to keep the thymus healthy and vital.

Pancreas

A healthy pancreas helps you properly digest the foods you eat, think more clearly, and maintain proper blood sugar levels in the body. The pancreas is both a digestive organ and an endocrine gland. It is found behind the lower part of the stomach, directly beneath the left lung. Elongated and tapered, it stretches about eight inches long across the back of the abdomen.

Digestively, the pancreas produces pancreatic juices that contain enzymes. These enzymes are first collected in the pancreatic duct and then released into the intestine to help metabolize carbohydrates, fats, and proteins. Its digestive secretions are important in neutralizing stomach acids. Hormonally, the endocrine tissue of the pancreas secretes insulin and glucagons that regulate the level of glucose (sugar) in the blood. Insulin, which is the most important of the pancreatic hormones, helps carry glucose from the bloodstream into our body's tissues and cells. When our body is producing just the right amount, our blood sugar levels and metabolism support overall good health. An adequate amount of glucose supports the proper working of our brains. Abnormal glucose levels, seen in diabetes, can damage the kidneys, eyes, blood vessels, and nerves. Inflammation of the pancreas can be either acute or chronic in nature, and pancreatic cancer is one of the most severe forms of malignancy.

Take care of your pancreas and it will care for you! Send lots of love and appreciation to your pancreas and thank it for helping your metabolism and for maintaining the proper level of sugar in your blood.

Ovaries

A healthy balance of ovarian hormones promotes a calm, clear mind, restful sleep, strong bones, healthy skin, vibrant energy, and sexual vitality.

The ovaries are paired glands that resemble unshelled almonds in both size and shape. Located in the pelvic cavity, the ovaries are responsible for the fluctuation of our hormone levels as women as well as the health of our sexual organs. The ovaries and their interaction with the pituitary and hypothalamus determine when, where, and how we have menstrual periods or deliver babies. After the ovaries' egg-producing phase ends, women come to the end of their fertile years. When we are no longer ovulating, our bodies slow down production of estrogen and our periods stop altogether.

It's important to note that making babies is not the only reason your ovaries exist. Ovaries are more than just egg sacs. They are endocrine organs that continually produce hormones before, during, and *after* menopause. After menopause, a woman's production of estrogen and progesterone drops dramatically but our ovaries continue to make androgens, the so-called male hormones like testosterone, though usually at lowered levels. Helpfully for women, these androgens get converted into estrogen in fat cells.

So, while hormone levels change dramatically as we age, those changes don't have to lead to a decrease in vitality, strength, and sexiness. Paying careful attention to diet and fitness, maintaining a healthy amount of muscle and fat, and keeping our energy flowing in our ovaries by using practices such as qigong will allow for continued vigor and zest in our lives. Contrary to popular belief, the menopausal ovary is neither failing nor useless. It is simply shifting from its function from reproduction to maintenance.

No matter what your age or point on the life cycle, as you emit qi to your ovaries, feel how juicy you are as a woman. With love and attention, we allow our ovaries to take good care of us for the whole of our lives.

Adrenals

Our adrenal glands carry us through stressful times in our lives, strengthening our immune system, boosting energy levels, and keeping our minds clear.

The adrenals are small, triangular glands located on top of both of your kidneys. Your adrenal glands are made of two parts that perform two very separate functions. One, the outer region called the adrenal cortex, produces sex hormones as well as hormones that regulate metabolism of fats, protein, and carbohydrates, and balance fluids. These hormones have an effect on the levels of sugar and minerals in the blood, immune system function, and blood pressure. The other, inner region of the adrenals, called the adrenal medulla, helps you cope with physical and emotional stress.

The adrenal cortex produces hormones that keep many of the body's processes in balance. The most well-known of these hormones is cortisol. This hormone has many effects including priming the body for fight and flight during stress, raising blood glucose levels, and reducing all types of inflammation. An appropriate amount of cortisol in the body is essential. When cortisol levels are elevated or decreased, serious health consequences arise.

The adrenal medulla secretes hormones such as epinephrine which increase heart rate, force heart contractions, facilitate blood flow to muscles and the brain, govern relaxation of muscles, and control asthma and allergies. The medulla also secretes norepinephrine, which affects muscles, metabolic processes, blood pressure control, cardiac output, and stress response. The adrenal medulla affects the sympathetic nervous system, which mobilizes our resources for action, responds to stimuli, and gets us ready and moving.

According to Chinese medicine, the sympathetic nervous system is a yang element. Yin, on the other hand, can be seen as a quality of the parasympathetic nervous system and the adrenal cortex, which govern the more inner world of nutrition, maintenance, and storage. Yin/yang balance within the adrenals is essential.

Chinese medicine conceives of the kidneys and adrenals as one. Healthy kidneys and adrenals are of utmost importance for a long and healthy life.

Properly functioning adrenal glands maintain a peaceful, tranquil state as well as peak immunity. So many of our life habits wreak havoc with our adrenals, promoting high levels of stress, nervous tension, and continuous fight-or-flight responses. Cultivating and nurturing the kidney, or adrenal energy, is of utmost importance in Chinese medicine, especially when it comes to being ageless.

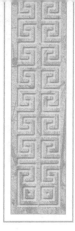

Strong Bones

In Set 6 we focus our mind intent further, shifting focus from the endocrine glands to the bones and taking the time to care for these remarkable structures so crucial to long, healthy lives.

SET 6: KNITTING STRONG BONES

Qigong exercises to maintain strong bones and good balance are called Bone Marrow Washing. These exercises were developed simultaneously with two other qigong forms. One is the muscle tendon classic done to maintain strong tendons and muscles, of which several are included in the Twenty-Minute Workout such as Phoenix Eats Its Ashes and Tigress Crouches Down. (The third system, eighteen Luohan Qigong has not been included in this book.) Bone-marrow-washing exercises date back to at least the sixth century A.D., when an Indian monk named Da Mo brought Buddhist teachings to China. On his visit to the now famous Shaolin Monastery, he found the monks sickly from long hours spent sitting in meditation. Da Mo created these exercises to develop flexibility and bone health, helping the monks heal their muscles, tendons, and marrow. This was the first time that meditation and martial arts were brought together as a unified system.

The purpose of the Bone Marrow Washing exercises was and is to promote qi and blood flow in the bones, in turn bringing oxygen to the bone marrow. Because the practice has always been closely linked with meditation, Bone Marrow Washing is also said to promote peace of mind and spiritual enlightenment.

Indeed, in addition to health, the two most significant benefits from these exercises are longevity and enhanced spiritual life. Bone Marrow Washing prevents aging of the joints and bones by bringing together the body and the mind. As we perform Bone Marrow Washing, we are indeed "washing" the red and white blood cells produced in our marrow which become "dirty" with age, or less effective at the same time the marrow becomes more fatty. But besides purifying our bodies, Bone Marrow Washing purifies our spirit. These exercises teach you how to regulate qi within the meridians and organs. The training encourages qi circulation to the bone and brain in particular, nourishing them and maintaining their proper function. When qi flows to the brain, it sparks the spirit.

Bone Marrow Washing exercises combine self-massage, mental concentration to direct qi, and breath control. As you practice, you expel pathogens from the bones and improve blood circulation, maximize qi flow, and increase flexibility. Washing the marrow provides you with the same kind of fresh healthy blood you had as a child. As the "mother of qi," the blood in Chinese medicine nourishes all the organs to bring you youthful vitality.

The qigong exercises in this set build bone mass in different ways. For one, these qigong exercises strengthen the kidneys, and the kidneys nourish the bones. Invigorating the kidney energy of the body balances and strengthens the hormonal system and thus the bones. Secondly, moving muscles and using weights stresses the bones, increasing bone mass. Our major muscles are attached to underlying bone by tendons. Every time a muscle contracts, it exerts a force on the bone to which it is anchored. The bone responds by building mass. Finally, the visualizations in this set help to infuse the marrow with energy, regenerating body and spirit.

PLAYING QI BALL

Weight-bearing exercise such as those in Playing Qi Ball are crucial for making and maintaining strong bones. Adding weights to your qigong movements helps to maintain bone integrity. When the muscles work harder, they in turn exert force on the bones, which stimulates the bones' natural ability to regenerate.

All things in moderation, though! Be careful not to lift too heavy a weight because too much weight can cause muscles to become pumped up, restricting the flow of qi.

Lifting Qi Ball

In addition to strengthening the bones, this exercise increases flexibility of shoulders and neck, promotes weight management, benefits lungs and heart, reduces stress and panic, promotes coordination, and treats headaches and neck problems.

As you do this exercise, you may experience a strong sensation of qi. In this exercise, the longer you move, the more you relax. Everything becomes easy and more harmonized. Think of yourself proudly offering the qi ball to the world as a precious gift.

Spinning Wheel

In addition to strengthening the bones through weight bearing this exercise tonifies the spleen, circulates and moves qi to the hands, smoothes qi in your entire body, disperses liver qi stagnation, promotes unrestrained flow of liver and gallbladder qi, treats digestive problems, and relieves constipation.

Notice how this exercise brings you in tune with the present moment. Feel the rhythm of your existence. Feel the beauty that makes you who you are. Feel your personal power.

VARIATION ‖ Speed up the tempo of this movement if you like. This will allow the centrifugal force to carry you along. Moving faster is fun and releases pent-up anger or frustration from your body. After you've moved quickly, slow things down again to experience the difference.

Back Swinging Monkey

When this exercise is done with qi balls it strengthens your bones. Practiced with or without the qi balls this exercise nurtures the heart and spirit, balances the mind, and calms the nerves. By opening both yin and yang energies of the arms, it lowers high blood pressure, promotes free and unrestrained flow of energy, combats fatigue, and helps with weight management.

By stimulating and opening the important gallbladder and liver meridians, Back Swinging Monkey relieves a variety of symptoms associated with these organs, including migraines, joint pain, and symptoms that accompany menopause. By twisting your body along its vertical axis, you release energy blockages, dispersing qi within your liver and gallbladder meridians on the sides of your body. The free flow of qi in these meridians in turn promotes the proper functioning of the spleen, heart, kidneys, stomach, and lungs.

As you increase the strength and flexibility of the muscles around the neck, you provide yourself with a wonderful antidote to the hunched posture that too often accompanies aging.

This exercise brings with it a tremendous lightness of being. It is free flowing and yet directs you where you need to go, providing the ease and focus needed to accomplish life tasks.

BONE-MARROW WASHING

The combination of breath and visualization in this exercise creates a balance of yin and yang in the body. This balances the female and male aspects and water and fire elements within your system. The exercise also:

stimulates production of red and white blood cells in the marrow
prevents illness
prevents symptoms of aging, such as wrinkles, gray hair, and hair loss
revitalizes skin

As you do the exercise, keep your inhalations and exhalations deep and coordinated with your movements. Let your mind and movements be calm

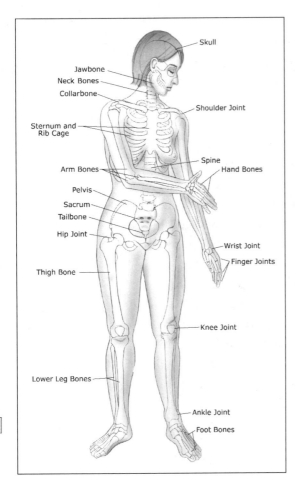

- Skull
- Jawbone
- Neck Bones
- Collarbone
- Shoulder Joint
- Sternum and Rib Cage
- Spine
- Arm Bones
- Hand Bones
- Pelvis
- Sacrum
- Tailbone
- Hip Joint
- Wrist Joint
- Finger Joints
- Thigh Bone
- Knee Joint
- Lower Leg Bones
- Ankle Joint
- Foot Bones

● *Skeletal System*

but energized. Inhale and visualize the qi going deep through your skin into the marrow of your bones.

Bringing in Earthly Waters

Water has a tremendous healing power, is thought to have a feminine quality, and, combined with fire, forms the basis of all life. As you do this exercise, imagine in detail the qualities of water that attract you, from its amazing force to its soothing properties. Maybe you love lakes, waterfalls, or the ocean. Image the water you love flowing swiftly downward as it cools you, showering and nurturing your yin aspects.

As women, we have a natural tendency toward yin, but often have yang excess in certain organs as well. When water and fire in the body are regulated properly, yin and yang will be in harmony. Inhaling builds water in the body because as you inhale you lead qi inward to the bone marrow, where water is stored. This reduces the qi in the muscles and tendons and calms the yang of the body.

The mind impacts whether the body is yin or yang. When the mind is regulated, so too is the breath. And when the breath is regulated, the mind can be calm. Without getting us too excited, which would create an imbalance of yang, qigong balances yin and yang and raises our spirits.

Spirit, known as *shen*, governs your qi to properly regulate water and fire in your body. Breath is sometimes called spirit breath because it is the vehicle for *shen*. As you become more aware of your *shen* during the exercise of Bringing in the Earthly and Heavenly Waters, you may feel that your spirit is breathing for you.

Bringing in Heavenly Fire

Like water, fire has purifying powers. Representing the active male yang principle, fire purges toxins. It melts, burns, liquefies, and transforms matter. Compared to other elements, fire stands alone in its ability to transform matter and change the underlying nature of all substances—perfect for creating strong, healthy bones!

As you bring in Heavenly Fire, visualize the energy coming from above and into your bones like the rays of the sun you soak in at the beach. Imagine your bones as plants, growing strong thanks to the nourishment of the sun. As you warm yourself with heavenly fire, you may feel as if fire is shooting out of your hands.

Fire provides the energy for human life, bringing light, warming the body, and increasing yang. It represents the burning desire of love, the spark that makes things happen, and the excitement of life. Fire strengthens your bones, bringing in warmth, promoting transformation, removing impurities, and melting away the unwanted fat developing in bones as we age.

The skeleton is the structure of your life. It is not only holding you up, but holding you together. It allows you to move from one place to the other without falling apart, and provides you with flexibility. By nourishing the bones in your skeleton with the life-enhancing qualities of fire, you will move through your life with certainty and conviction.

Mixing Fire and Water

Together, water and fire make up the essential elements necessary to adequately nourish our bones. Made up of oxygen and hydrogen, water needs the spark of fire in order for both its gases to combine.

While we all need the spark of life that yang provides, when there is a predominance of yang, the body degenerates and ages because it is being burned out. Bringing water in with your inhalation to cool your body slows the degeneration process, allowing you to live a longer and healthier life. Exhaling creates more fire because it brings qi out toward the muscles, tendons, and skin where yang belongs, and energizes these areas. To release excess yang from your body, visualize the healthy mixing of the fire and water within.

Place your hand over your middle *dantian*. Due to its proximity to your heart and pericardium, which are fire organs according to the law of the five elements, this brings you in touch with the fire within. Place your other hand over your lower *dantian*. This relates to water because of its proximity to the kidneys, which are water element organs.

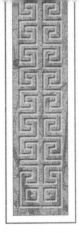

Energy, Spirit, Essence

THE FINAL set in the workout creates a long-lasting abundance not only of qi, but of the substances known as *shen,* or spirit, and *jing,* or essence. Together, qi, *shen,* and *jing* are known as the Three Treasures. Healthy amounts of each are essential to the ageless woman.

SET 7: NOURISHING THREE TREASURES

The Three Treasures are crucial to human existence. We need all three of the treasures to enjoy excellent health. Qi, or vital energy, is the force that animates life and all biological processes. *Shen,* or spirit, is the mind and the seat of consciousness. *Jing,* or essence, consists of hormones, reproductive, saliva, vaginal lubrication, ova, menstrual blood (semen and sperm in men), and other body fluids. It is the source of sexual maturation, reproduction, and growth of the body.

A major tenet of traditional Chinese medicine is the belief that people are born with the Three Treasures, which are fostered with healthy food and exercise. The Three Treasures are intimately related to the aging process. Cultivating these treasures and understanding how they affect the functioning of the body is essential to our well-being, helping us to make sound, healthy choices in our life.

The exercise in Set 7 balances, cleanses, and unifies all Three Treasures by smoothing scattered qi, creating ample flow of blood, promoting a plentiful supply of *jing* within the body, and calming and nourishing the *shen*.

Lady Raises Lotus to the Temple

As you do this exercise, you invigorate your supply of each of the Three Treasures in the three *dantian*s where they are stored. The upper *dantian* cultivates and stores the *shen*. The middle *dantian* cultivates and stores the qi. The lower *dantian* cultivates and stores the *jing*. As you move the lotus upward in this exercise, you enliven the Three Treasures in all three *dantian*s.

It is traditionally believed that people are endowed with different amounts of the treasures, but most are born with an abundant supply. A fundamental relationship is believed to exist between the three. An accumulation of one, in turn, creates abundance in another. A person's lifestyle and habits determine how these innate treasures are cultivated and preserved, which in turn effects the length and quality of their lives.

This exercise gathers, cleanses, and balances the Three Treasures. The lotus represents the combined and refined Three Treasures. The temple represents the heavenly and divine. The end result of bringing the lotus to the temple is a clear and peaceful mind, a strong and focused will, and a body filled with health and longevity—truly an experience of heaven on earth.

Qi (Vital Energy)

The most widely known of the Three Treasures is qi (vital energy), which refers to the life force flowing throughout every cell and tissue of the body. It is the motivator, the mover of all vital functions and transformations in the human body. Life is sustained as long as qi exists. Without qi, we die. The source of qi after birth comes from food, water, herbs, and air, which are digested and eventually transformed into qi.

During the slow and rhythmical movements of qigong, one's breath is used to cultivate vital energy, which further affects the *shen*. Qigong also calms the emotions, balances energy, and creates an experience of openness and peace. This creates a free flow not only of qi, but also blood, which invigorates the body's organs, stimulates glands, and tones other vital tissues. Blood is the substance most responsible for transporting nourishment, thus supporting the welfare of the physical body.

Shen (Spirit)

Shen represents all aspects of consciousness and mind. This includes awareness and cognition, thought and feeling, and will and intent. All of these aspects are reflected in one's personality. A combination of flexibility, spontaneity, and freedom from judgment is a way to achieve a healthy *shen*. The more your mind flows, the more your qi will flow.

Jing (Essence)

Jing determines genetic makeup because it forms the initial substance from which the body is created. There is the *jing* we are born with, derived from our parents, and the *jing* we cultivate during our lives as nourishment derived from the food and water we ingest after birth. The quality of our *jing* determines longevity and resistance to disease. If strong, we lead a long life, free of degenerative disease. Weak *jing* manifests in adults as premature aging. Tooth decay, arthritis, osteoporosis, and senility are all examples of the physical and mental deterioration that occur with diminishing *jing*.

Our bodies have a finite amount of *jing* at birth. When it's used up, we die. Fortunately, there exists another form of *jing*, which accumulates from energy left over at the end of a day. This energy is then transformed during sleep and is used to protect our *jing* from being consumed too quickly. As we age, unless we find ways of restoring *jing*, we normally don't produce as much excess energy and consequently use up our essence more quickly.

Cultivation of the Three Treasures creates peace of mind. One of the most famous qigong sayings is "refine the *jing* to create qi, refine qi to create *shen*, refine *shen* and return to the Void." The Void here refers to a clear and empty mind.

Creating and maintaining vibrant health and strength of the physical body can best be accomplished by protecting *jing*, raising *shen*, making qi and blood abundant, and training the muscles, tendons, and bones. Combined with the rest of the Twenty-Minute Workout, this set cultivates the Three Treasures as it brings them closer to their original state of abundance. In this way, we prevent disease and degeneration, retard the aging process, and prolong our lives.

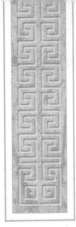

Storing Qi

THE TWENTY-MINUTE workout has generated and directed a tremendous amount of energy in your body. As you prepare to end your workout and turn to other things, it is important to first smooth and then store the qi you have cultivated so you may draw upon it as you go about your daily life. The warm-down helps you do just that.

WARM-DOWN

The purpose of the final part of the Twenty-Minute Workout is to release any remaining blockages in qi, to consolidate and store the qi you have generated in previous sets, and to create a gentle transition back to your normal state of being.

Mini Yin Massage

A simple technique that can be practiced anywhere, anytime, this massage regenerates the muscles and helps them to hold more blood. It provides additional nourishment to the tissues so they grow stronger. People from all cultures have instinctively performed therapeutic massage to help relieve sore muscles and facilitate speedy recovery from injury. The physical manipulation of the soft tissues of the body is also an effective treatment for many common ailments.

Massage can relieve headaches, joint pain, and stomach discomfort, in addition to strengthening weakened organs. It regulates the qi and blood circulating in your body, loosening and relaxing muscles along the qi pathways.

Chinese massage is performed by lightly rubbing the skin over meridians, acupoints, organs, muscles, and joints. It is most beneficial after you have felt, moved, cultivated, and stored qi during your qigong workout.

As you perform massage, you press and stimulate the endings of the nerves and qi channels located on the hands and feet and other parts of the body. When you rub in a way that creates friction, this limbers up joints, tendons, and muscles and facilitates the removal of deposits by breaking wastes down in the body. It also helps reduce swelling after nerve inflammation. Massage helps you clear your mind and eliminate stagnant qi that can remain in certain pockets of the body and cause pain.

SUGGESTIONS ‖

Hands: Before you begin, rub the center of the palm with the thumb, stimulating *laogong.* By massaging this point, you also gently stimulate the heart.

Knees: To warm the knees and relieve stiffness, use the open hand to rub around the whole joint.

Head: Massage the scalp to create build-up of qi throughout the head.

Feet: Rub the center of the bottoms of your feet with your thumb. This stimulates the kidneys via the Bubbling Well point, the first point on the kidney meridian.

Joints: Stiff and swollen joints, sprains, and bruises can be alleviated by self-massage. Gentle stroking and kneading is recommended on and around the injured tissues. But if you have severe joint injuries, consult your physician first.

Scalp: Comb your hair vigorously back with your fingers as you massage your scalp, stimulating the bladder, gallbladder, stomach, and triple warmer meridians for relief from high blood pressure, problems with the eyes, and to improve blood flow to the brain.

Feathering

This motion relieves congestion or pain, consolidates and conserves personal energy, and dispels negative energy others bring to us. It smoothes the qi stimulated and cultivated throughout the practice, readying it for storage in the *dantian*.

The fingertips sweep down the energy field that exists on the surface of our skin as if brushing away pain. With gentle, flowing movements and barely touching your own skin, you "dust off" and smooth the energy field that emanates from and surrounds your body.

> **Helpful Hint**
> Brush toward an imaginary line running up the center of your body if tired, weak, or depleted. Brush away from this centerline if you feel tense or are in pain.

Drinking Divine Water

This exercise strengthens and prevents aging of the joints and bones and promotes healthy teeth by stimulating their roots, creating saliva to kill germs in the mouth, to prevent tooth decay. The exercise activates digestion and prevents digestive problems by creating more saliva to break food down prior to reaching the stomach. It soothes the heart and clears the mind by causing vibrations in the skull.

After every qigong exercise, you may choose to bring the qi back to your *dantian* by swallowing your saliva. This exercise also opens the conception vessel, nourishes internal organs, and strengthens the connections between the conception and governing vessels, the important yin and yang meridians that run up the front and back of your body and create a circuit that connects and balances energy in your whole being.

Storing Body Qi

It's very important to end any qigong practice by storing the energy in the navel. The area around the navel can safely handle the increased energy generated by the qigong movements.

After Storing Body Qi, create a unification of the energy in your entire body. Feel the fullness of your energy by connecting your upper *dantian* (Sea of Spirit), your middle *dantian* (Sea of Tranquility), and your lower *dantian* (Sea of Energy). This creates a protective shield between you and the outside world, closing the circle of energy. In this way, excess energy moved during your practice doesn't disperse or leak out. By consolidating qi in your lower *dantian,* you ensure that it doesn't remain in your head or heart areas, but concentrates in your healing reserve, where you can use it to combat stress and negative influences from outside.

Creating friction between your hands at the end of your workout is a good way of consolidating your qi in the hands, which can then be used to emit qi. As you rub, push your palms together, creating heat and stimulating the entry of the qi into your hands. Focus your attention on the *laogong* points located on your palms and also concentrate on your fingertips.

Your hands are both the receivers and transmitters of energy. The *laogong* point is like a spring that connects the underground rivers of the lung, heart, and pericardium meridians. It is not only used to emit qi, but also connects your qi with the outer world. You may think of your qi both as breath that is drawn in from the natural world by your lungs and as loving energy that, through the pericardium meridian, radiates from the heart and its casing down through your hands and back out into the world again through *laogong*. The tips of your fingers, especially the index finger and the middle finger (which is the end point of the pericardium meridian), can transmit qi quite effectively. When these two fingers are joined together, they form a strong seal. This seal can then be used to transmit qi to parts of your body that may need extra attention after your workout.

Finally, as the qigong saying goes, "replace ten thousand thoughts with one thought." If you do this your energy will flow like an endless river, replenishing every aspect of your life.

Healing the Root

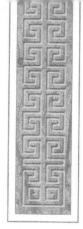

The Many Faces of Qi

By now you are quite familiar with the all-important concept of qi. You have felt its movement throughout your own body as you followed the workout in Part One. In Part Two, you learned of other concepts underlying qigong practice, such as yin and yang, meridians, the five elements, *shen* and *jing,* and blood, that interact with your qi to create overall health and fitness. On different days during your practice, you may have noticed your qi "behaving" differently. And if you have experienced any of the common symptoms I describe below, you certainly know that your qi can show many faces.

Just as the indigenous people of the Arctic are said to have hundreds of words for snow, practitioners of Chinese medicine have many different ways to describe qi. And why not? The Chinese have been closely observing qi in action for centuries. Although it cannot usually be seen, there can be no doubt of qi's effect in the body. Qi "acts" in different ways at different times. In patient after patient, the range of symptoms created by qi's behavior has informed traditional Chinese medicine practitioners about qi's qualities. A number of different qualities and patterns of qi have been observed. Some of these are:

stagnant qi—when qi is not moving smoothly, gets stuck, and is thus too abundant in certain parts of the body, resulting in pain or organ impairment, injuries, distention, and inflammation.

deficient qi—when there is not enough qi in the body, resulting in weakness and fatigue.

rebellious qi—when qi is going in the wrong direction, as when it rises up and out of the body in a condition such as vomiting or hiccups.

collapsed qi—when qi is so deficient it can no longer hold internal organs in their place.

Usually, these patterns and others show up in a complex of symptoms, which stem from imbalance in the organs. For example, a person with stagnant liver qi may complain of pain and swelling in the breasts, and have deep anger. Deficient heart qi may result in a weak pulse, excessive fatigue, and palpitations. Blood, *shen,* and *jing* may also be deficient or stagnant in an organ, causing a variety of symptoms. Also, organs are often described as having too much yang, too little yin, or vice versa. Qigong gets to the root of your symptom by balancing qi, *shen, jing,* and blood, and the forces of yin and yang within you.

Chinese medicine also ascribes sickness to outside influences from nature that create patterns of disharmony, such as too much dampness, cold, dryness, fire, or wind. Another type of influence called "pestilential factors" come from the outside in the form of viruses and bacteria which can wreak havoc with one's physical health. There are emotional influences that can have adverse effects on the physical body. All of these outside influences can have a deleterious effect on the body's qi and can manifest in illness.

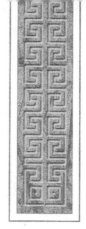

Healthy Relationships

QIGONG helps you build healthy relationships: between you and your body, between the yin and yang energies in your body, between the five natural elements that compose your being, between your organs, between you and others, and between you, nature, and the cosmos.

Qigong is an ancient practice that stems from a very complex culture. At first, the traditional Chinese way of viewing the body seems so different from what many of us are used to. But when you delve into it, you find it really makes sense. When it comes to treating illness with qigong, practitioners of Chinese medicine utilize a holistic approach; they look for patterns in the body and assess the state of their patient's emotions, physical conditions, and mental and spiritual state.

As you consult this guide to your symptoms, know that your body is a complex landscape. The treatments I suggest below are for the most prevalent patterns I see in my acupuncture practice. There are other organ systems that may come into the picture for you. Realize that the explanations below are not exhaustive. Your landscape is unique.

What works for one person may not work for another. You will need to use your intuition and observation of how your body responds to treatment in determining which patterns you may have. You may choose to consult a practitioner of traditional Chinese medicine such as an acupuncturist for evaluation. All of the treatments described below, however, are simple and easy to do yourself and can do no harm.

THE FIVE ELEMENTS AND YOUR ORGANS

As you know, the Chinese traditionally believe that all of nature, including our bodies and the organs inside of us, are made up of yin and yang and the five elements of fire, earth, metal, water, and wood. The relationships between these elements—how they affect each other—have an enormous effect on the health and fitness of our bodies (see five elements illustration page 95). The five elements are connected through the Nurturing (*shen*) Cycle and the Controlling (*ko*) Cycle. Traditionally, the grandparent is said to be the controller and the mother is the nurturer; however, I have substituted the father for the grandparent for our Western context.

There is an interrelationship between each of the five elements via the organ systems associated with them. In this way of looking at the body one organ system both nurtures and is at the same time controlled or "quelled" by another organ system. This means that each organ system has multiple effects on other organs in the system and vice versa. For example, just as water quells fire it is also fed by metal; just as fire quells metal it is fed by wood; and just as metal quells (or cuts) wood it is also fed by earth, and so on and so forth.

You can also think of this system as a family of sorts whereby each organ is a family member in relation to another organ. In its role of "mother," an organ nurtures the organ that is its "child." In its role as "father," each organ controls the organ that is its "child." As discussed in Part Two, each organ also has a sister (or brother) organ (yang organs have a yin counterpart and vice versa). By balancing the flow of energy through the five-element cycle, qigong makes sure all our organs in the family that is our body receive the nurturing and management they need.

The five-element theory is a model for how to create and maintain balance and health within the person as a whole. In Chinese medicine, we do not usually treat individual organs or symptoms without considering the rest of the body. We treat the whole family. This is both figuratively and literally true.

When a child is brought into my office for treatment, not only do I examine the interrelationship of all the child's symptoms, I look to the parents who bought him in. For example, the child may be suffering from poor digestion. He looks pale and is tired, overweight, retaining water, and complaining of sore muscles. He is unhappy and unable to make decisions. In this case I would suspect a deficiency of spleen qi. But how does one treat the spleen according to the five elements?

According to the five elements, the "mother" heart (fire element) nourishes the "child" spleen (earth element) and "father" liver (wood element) controls the "child" spleen. In other words, the spleen is both nourished by the heart, its mother, and controlled by the liver, its father. More often than not, in the case of the child with deficient spleen qi, I would also notice that the mother is distraught, self-consumed, and not able to nurture and nourish her child. She represents a heart out of balance. The father, on the other hand, may be angry and belligerent and so out of control in his own life that he has little control over his child. He represents an imbalance of liver energy. In this case, I would treat the parents in order to treat the child, in other words treating the heart and liver in addition to treating the spleen. I might also look to the child's siblings (sister or brother organs), who have an intimate and direct effect on how the child feels and behaves. The sister organ in this case would be the stomach.

Clearly, the organs in our bodies are intimately interrelated and profoundly affect each other just as members of a family do. When one organ over-controls or saps energy from another, practicing qigong restores balance among and between the organs and thus the five elements.

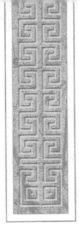

Getting to the Point

IN THIS PART, I recommend a variety of treatments to address twenty-five symptoms of particular concern for women. These treatments include: qigong exercises from the workout and a few new ones to target certain illness patterns, recommendations for lifestyle and dietary changes, and a greater focus on acupoints.

Self-acupressure has always been an important part of qigong. As an acupuncturist, I see the remarkable effects of acupoint stimulation on a daily basis. For these reasons, I have paid special attention to instructing you on the powerful art of self-acupressure. Unlike acupuncture, acupressure requires no in-depth training . . . and no needles! Safe and easy, it can be highly effective for treating and preventing both symptoms and their root causes. It's also great for the general purposes of increasing circulation, dissolving tension and stress, relieving pain, and boosting immunity.

HOW TO DO SELF-ACUPRESSURE

Give yourself acupressure anytime, anywhere, as a preventive measure for overall good health, treatment for a chronic illness, or first-aid for a symptom that comes on suddenly.

For the purposes of prevention and treatment of illness, I recommend that you practice self-acupressure in a quiet place where you can concentrate on your breathing and achieve a relaxed, receptive state of mind and body.

Use the illustrations and pictures to help you find the points. Know that every body is unique and your point may not correspond exactly to the point on the illustration or picture. Acupoints are usually located on "anatomical landmarks"—high or low places on the body, under muscle groups or in a muscle, and near or between bones. You will even be able to feel some points as slight indentations on your skin.

You will know the acupoint when you find it! When pressed, it will be a little more tender than other spots around it. You should experience a "good hurt" and this will tell you that you've hit your mark.

Use firm pressure on the point. You may choose to use your thumb, middle finger, heel of the hand, or side of the hand. Each method has its merits, and you are free to choose the one you like best. Try pressing the point with a smooth, hard object such as a pointed stone with a rounded tip. You can do this as a variation or if uncomfortable using your fingers due to joint pain, for instance. Apply pressure gradually, avoiding abrupt, forceful pressure.

Be gentle in sensitive areas, such as around lymph nodes (see lymphatic system illustration page 91), and avoid areas where you have injuries to your skin. Be especially careful with acupoints on your abdomen. If you are pregnant or seriously ill, consult your physician before performing self-acupressure.

In general, do self-acupressure no more than once a day and for no more than an hour at a time. If you are in generally good health, once or twice a week should suffice. Press each point for about a minute, and not more than two. Become aware of the way the pressure influences your qi. With time and practice, you will be able to feel when it is time to stop the pressure.

The following section contains illustrations with all of the points recommended in this part. There are also photographs of select acupoints on the legs, feet, arms and hands. These have been included so that you can get a real feel of what it looks like to do acupressure on yourself. It also helps you to see the location, not just from a drawing but on the body itself. You can do one or all of the following acupoint recommendations for your specific condition or symptom. Make sure to press the point on both sides of your body. You will definitely feel the difference! What follows is an overview of the acupressure points that will be discussed in this section. Use this section as a reference for the recommendations in this part.

INNER LEG ACUPOINTS

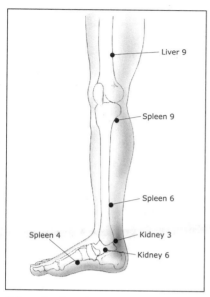

● Inner Leg Acupoints

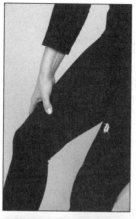

● *Liver 9: Located on both legs, four inches above the inner, upper corner of your knee cap slightly toward the inner thigh.*

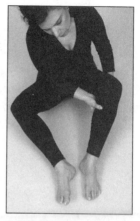

● *Spleen 9: Located on each leg, tucked underneath the inner side of your knee and the big bone on your inner leg.*

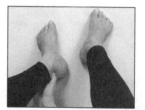

● *Kidney 3: On each foot behind the inner ankle bone midway between this bone and the Achilles tendon.*

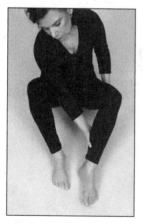

● *Spleen 6: Three inches above each ankle bone on the inner part of your lower leg, in the depression behind the big bone there.*

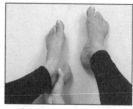

● *Kidney 6: On each foot in the depression underneath the center of the inner ankle bone.*

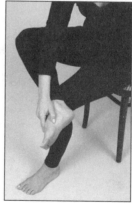

● *Spleen 4: One inch behind the joints of each big toe, on the first metatarsal bone, which is the long bone between the big toe and the ankle.*

OUTER LEG ACUPOINTS

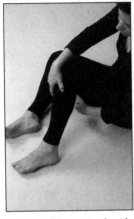

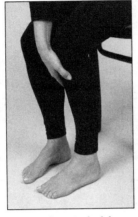

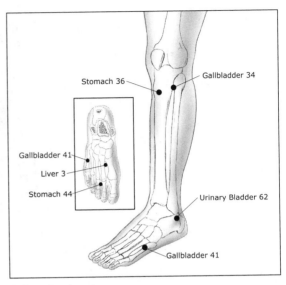

● *Gallbladder 34: On the side of each lower leg in a depression found in the juncture of the two bones of the leg.*

● *Stomach 36: On both legs, about 3 inches below the center of your knee cap and one inch out from the edge of the leg bone.*

● *Outer Leg Acupoints*

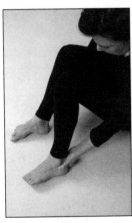

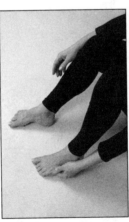

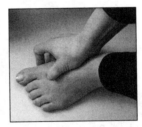

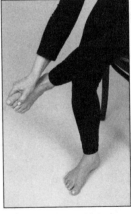

● *Urinary Bladder 62: On both feet about a half an inch directly down from the bottom of the outer ankle bone.*

● *Gallbladder 41: On the top of both feet in a depression where the fourth toe and the baby toe meet.*

● *Liver 3: On the tops of both feet about two inches from the web of the big toe and the second toe, in between the meeting point of the bones of these two toes.*

● *Stomach 44: On the top side of each foot one-eighth of an inch from the web between the second and third toes.*

OUTER ARM ACUPOINTS

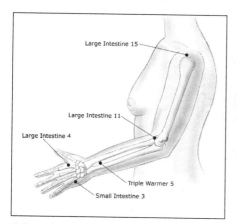

Large Intestine 15

Large Intestine 11

Large Intestine 4

Triple Warmer 5

Small Intestine 3

● *Outer Arm Acupoints*

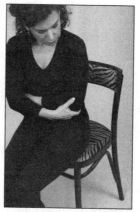

● *Large Intestine 11: On both elbows, in a depression where the bones of the lower and upper arms meet. Find with arm bent at right angle on the inner side of the joint.*

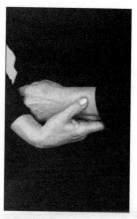

● *Triple Warmer 5: On both arms, two inches above both wrists in the center of the arm.*

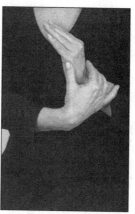

● *Small Intestine 3: On both hands, beneath the knuckle on your pinky finger.*

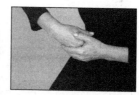

● *Large Intestine 4: On both hands, between the thumb and pointer finger, this point is located at the top of a mound created when your thumb is held right next to your pointer finger. Push against the middle of the bone located between the base of the pointer finger and the wrist.*

PALM SIDE OF WRIST ACUPOINTS

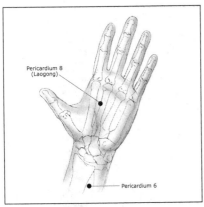

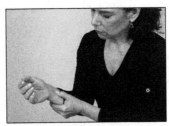

● Pericardium 6: On the palmar side each arm, two inches above the crease of your wrist and in between the two tendons.

● Palm Side of Wrist Acupoints

TORSO ACUPOINTS

Qigong for Staying Young

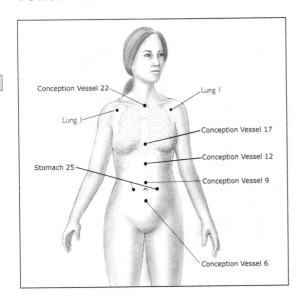

● Torso Acupoints

Lung 1: On each side of the upper chest, in the depression about an inch below the edge of the collarbone near the shoulder joint.

Conception Vessel 22: On the centerline of the torso in the depression above the sternum (breastbone) and between the collarbones.

Conception Vessel 17: Midway between the breasts, on the middle of the sternum (breastbone).

Conception Vessel 12: Halfway between Conception Vessel 17 and the navel.

Stomach 25: On both sides of the abdomen, about one inch to the side of the belly button.

Conception Vessel 9: Approximately one inch directly above the navel.

Conception Vessel 6: One and a half inches below belly button on midline of the body.

BACK OF HEAD ACUPOINTS

● *Back of Head Acupoints*

Gallbladder 20: On both sides, in the depression under the ridge at the bottom of your skull about an inch from the spine.

Hundred Meeting Point (Governing Vessel 20, Crown): On the top center of the head at the point where an imaginary line drawn from the tops of the ears would meet.

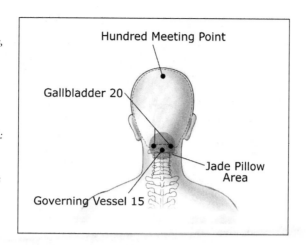

Hundred Meeting Point

Gallbladder 20

Jade Pillow Area

Governing Vessel 15

FACE ACUPOINTS

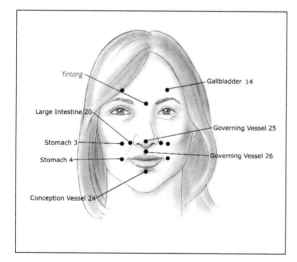

Yintang

Gallbladder 14

Large Intestine 20

Governing Vessel 25

Stomach 3

Governing Vessel 26

Stomach 4

Conception Vessel 24

● *Face Acupoints*

Yintang: *In the center of the forehead between the eyebrows.*

Large Intestine 20: *In a depression at the side of each nostril.*

Gallbladder 14: *Over each eye, about an inch above the center of the eyebrow.*

Stomach 3: *On both cheeks, in a depression level with the bottom of your nostril directly under the center of your eye.*

Stomach 4: *On both sides of your face, one quarter of an inch from the corner of the mouth.*

Governing Vessel 25: *On the tip of the nose.*

Governing Vessel 26: *In the depression on the center of the upper lip, where the upper teeth and gums meet.*

Conception Vessel 24: *Between the upper lip and nose, in the depression between the lower lip and bottom of your chin.*

SIDE OF FACE ACUPOINTS

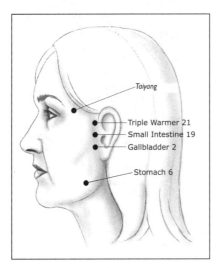

● *Side of Face Acupoints*

Taiyang: *On both sides of your face, on your temple, located about one inch behind the corner of your eye.*

Triple Warmer 21, Small Intestine 19, and Gallbladder 2: Three acupoints on both sides of the head, located in front of the ear about a quarter of an inch from where the ear meets the face. These points are found in the hollow formed when the mouth is open.

Stomach 6: On both sides of your face, on top of the bump of muscle formed at the corner of your jaws.

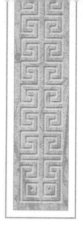

Anxiety and Palpitations

ANXIETY is one of the most common problems I see in my practice. Women in particular often worry about children, personal relationships, work, or finances. You may feel trapped, fear being alone, or fear that you won't be able to keep your life in order. Maybe you can't find humor in anything, or are just overwhelmed. Symptoms of anxiety include: a pit in your stomach, trouble falling asleep, waking up in the middle of the night with palpitations, sweating profusely for no reason, feeling disoriented, being excessively nervous, irritable, and fear-ridden, or experiencing chest heaviness and tightness. In extreme cases, you may also want to run for no apparent reason, be afraid to be left in a room with the door closed, avoid elevators, and have a sensation of your throat closing up, nausea, or shaking.

The practice of qigong calms us down and promotes the proper functioning of the parasympathetic nervous system, which brings us to a normal, balanced, and centered state of being. Many sufferers of anxiety will notice relief from their symptoms just by doing the Twenty-Minute Workout. If you need more help with anxiety, the key is in your breath. When you connect with your breathing during times of anxiety, this is often all you will need to be able to reverse symptoms. How do you "connect with your breathing"? It's really quite simple.

NURTURING HEART EXERCISE

First, during an anxiety attack, it's important not to get upset with yourself. Tell yourself to be patient and that your symptoms will soon go away. When you begin to experience symptoms, go to a space apart from others where you can find some peace and quiet. Choose a comfortable place to sit. Sit down and place your feet flat on the floor. Sit up straight and place your right hand on your chest (at your middle *dantian*). Place your left hand on your lower *dantian* and begin taking slow, deep breaths. Keep your eyes open and concentrate on your body expanding and contracting with each breath. With every breath, visualize your energy sinking lower and lower into your body. Do from one to three minutes.

It is believed that anxiety stems from disharmony between your kidneys and heart. This simple exercise centers you and creates harmony between these two organs. Placing your hand on your middle *dantian* nourishes and calms the energy of your heart, which "houses the mind." Placing your hand on your lower *dantian* nourishes the energy of your kidneys. The emotion of your kidneys is fear, the root of most anxiety attacks. When you strengthen the energy of your kidneys by breathing into your lower *dantian*, you release fear from your body. When doing this exercise, fill your body with a sense of security by telling yourself that everything is fine, you are safe, no one will hurt you, and there is no reason to run. See also Breathing into Beautiful Belly under "Breathing Difficulty" (page 177).

Many patients suffering from anxiety tell me they feel they are not in their skin. This common anxiety symptom occurs when qi rises upward and even out of your body and your heart is no longer providing a stable house for your mind. When you practice qigong, no matter what the exercise, concentrate on bringing your energy down to your lower *dantian*. Feel your feet being planted and connected to the earth. In doing so, you create a secure, solid physical vessel that holds you safe and sound, centered firmly within yourself.

● *Soothe Anxiety Exercise*

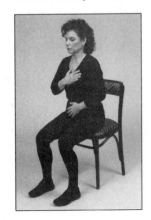

Woman Connects with Heaven and Earth reinforces the connection of heart and kidneys. Beautiful Woman Turns at Waist and Monkey Stretches Up and Down are excellent ways to further strengthen your kidney energy and alleviate fear. Lady Raises Lotus to the Temple helps with anxiety by working with the heart energy to pacify the spirit. A great support in troubled times, it also helps you to connect with yourself and open your heart up to others in a loving way.

Because prevention is half the cure, express and process your emotions on a regular basis. Allowing fear and worry to build up inside of you can damage your qi in the long run. Just as the earth sometimes gives off small tremors to release the pressure in its fault lines, you too, must release emotions gently and appropriately to avoid grand-scale emotional earthquakes and catastrophic health problems.

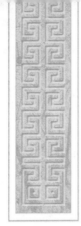

Arthritis, Muscular Problems, and Tendon Pain or Weakness

ARTHRITIS

From the viewpoint of Chinese medicine, pain in your joints is caused by a blockage of qi and blood. This blockage stems from coldness, wind, or dampness and is known as Bi syndrome, a condition similar to what Western medicine calls arthritis. It is no coincidence that arthritis sufferers run to warm, dry climates for relief. Keeping warm and dry and avoiding the wind is very important. It is also essential if you are suffering from joint pain that you get up and move. Just as a moving door hinge doesn't get rusty, joints that keep moving stay free of inflammation. Moderation is key, however. You don't want to traumatize your joints with excessive, high-impact exercise. Qigong, which promotes the flow of qi throughout the body and eliminates stagnant energy stuck in joints, is a perfect exercise for sufferers of joint pain. During your workout, you may choose to concentrate on exercises that release pain throughout your body, such as Fluffing White Clouds. Or you may do those exercises that gently move the parts of your body where you feel most pain:

- for the wrists, elbows, and hands, Flapping Wrists and Opening Qi Door
- for the shoulders, Separating Clouds and Spinning Wheel
- for the hips, Beautiful Woman Turns at Hips
- for knee and ankle pain, Circling Knees

To relieve joint pain, press gently on the following acupoints:

- Large Intestine 4 and Liver 3 done together release pain all over the body
- Gallbladder 20 combined with Large Intestine 4 to release pain that migrates from one place to another like the wind
- Spleen 9 to disperse pain caused by excessive dampness
- Triple Warmer 5 for pain of the fingers, elbows, upper back, and neck

To release stagnant energy in all joints and stiff areas of your body, practice Shaking the Tree. This is a spontaneous qigong exercise, meaning it has no exact form and you create it for yourself. It takes twenty to thirty seconds to do. Standing comfortably, simply shake your body out in any way you see fit. You may choose to shake out your legs, then your arms. You can shake both limbs together or one at a time. Shake out your upper body, then turn and shake out the tension in your neck and shoulders. Move in any way that you like, creating natural gyrations in certain areas, releasing your own unique blockages. You may feel a little silly if anyone happens to be watching you, but your joints will thank you later!

Avoid the application of ice to relieve pain in the body. The ice may give you temporary relief, but because arthritis is a cold/damp problem, by cutting

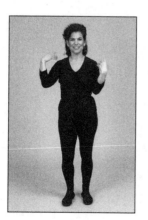 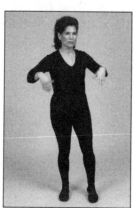

● *Shaking Tree*

off blood flow to the affected area, ice will eventually make your joint pain worse. Instead, use qigong and self-acupressure to open up the flow of energy to a specific body part or throughout the body. This brings fresh, clean, oxygenated new blood into the area to create healing and release pain.

Eat warm, dry foods to counteract the cold/damp condition. Choose cooked or baked dishes such as rice and other whole grains, vegetables, fish, poultry, tofu and other meat substitutes. Dried foods such as dehydrated fruits, seaweed, seeds, and nuts, are also good for people with joint pain. Avoid vegetables in the nightshade family such as tomatoes, potatoes, eggplant, and peppers. This includes all types of peppers and potatoes except sweet potatoes. These vegetables grow at night and thus are considered cold in nature. The Chinese also warn against eating citrus fruits because of their highly acidic, cold nature, said to cause arthritis, especially when eaten in great amounts after an operation or accident.

Sometimes the aching and pain in your joints makes an affected area feel more hot than cold. This heat can be a result of a severely deficient condition or a buildup of stagnant qi in the joints. You can tell if you have a hot problem if you feel heat emanating from your joints when you touch them, if they appear red and swollen, or if application of heat makes them feel worse. If you have a hot condition, it is particularly important to strengthen your system by eating a balanced, healthy diet. Avoid spicy foods, specifically green onions. Avoid alcohol and smoking. Practice the Healing Sounds for Kidney and Liver. As you inhale, visualize strong healing energy coming into your kidney and liver organs and when you exhale, see the excess heat leaving your body. This will nourish the yin (water) of your kidneys and liver and also release excess yang (fire) from your liver.

Do self-acupressure on:

- Kidney 6 and Kidney 3 to cool heat
- Gallbladder 34 to clear heat, promote free flowing energy, and strengthen tendons and bones
- Triple Warmer 5 to relieve hot conditions and release stagnant qi

If you suffer from osteoarthritis there is even more reason to strengthen the kidneys. It is beneficial to do the exercises in Set 6 for Knitting Strong Bones.

MUSCULAR PAIN

The spleen governs and strengthens our muscles and flesh. Eat naturally sweet yellow or orange foods such as yams and sweet potatoes, winter squashes, carrots, papaya, dates, brown rice, millet, oatmeal, sweet rice, and barley to nourish the spleen energy and consequently the muscles. When there is pain in the muscles, practice the following exercises:

- Swan Stretches Her Wings
- Healing Sound for Spleen
- Thump Pump
- Rag Doll Twist
- Mini Yin Massage

TENDON AND LIGAMENT PAIN

According to the principles of Chinese medicine, the liver governs and tones our ligaments and tendons. Our joints need the support of healthy ligaments and tendons nourished with ample blood: blood that comes from balanced liver energy. Alleviate pain by practicing the Healing Sound for Liver to release stagnant energy.

Do a liver cleanse in the morning to clear and cool the liver once or twice a month. This consists of drinking lemonade made from the juice of two lemons, a large dash of cayenne pepper, and a teaspoon of maple syrup. Wait one hour before eating your first food for the day. Remember not to overexercise with heavy aerobic training since it injures the liver and tendons. Eat red and purple grapes, a reputed Chinese nutritional remedy for the tendons. Eat more sour or green foods for the liver.

High-quality fresh oils are beneficial to the liver. Olive and flaxseed oils are particularly recommended. Eat a moderate amount of raw organic whole nuts and seeds. Choose organic butter over margarine.

Phoenix Eats Its Ashes and Tigress Crouches Down are muscle and tendon fortifying exercises.

LOW BACK PAIN

When it comes to pain, whether muscular, ligament and tendon, or bone-related, low back and neck pain are two of the most common complaints I hear from my female patients.

As with arthritis, the treatment for low back pain is to nourish and strengthen the kidneys. Low back pain is caused by a deficiency of the kidneys, disruption of qi flow in the urinary bladder meridian, wind, dampness, or external injury to the muscles of the lower back. The following exercises resolve the imbalances of the kidneys and help to strengthen the lower back:

- Kidney Rub for Life (page 103)
- Energize Endocrines for Adrenals
- Healing Sound for Kidneys
- Phoenix Eats Its Ashes
- Woman Connects with Heaven and Earth
- Monkey Stretches Up and Down
- Standing Like a Tree, Exercise 8

Also, while in Horse Stance (page 11), do self-acupressure on Small Intestine 3 and Governing Vessel 26 to treat the governing meridian that runs up the back.

NECK PAIN

Pain in your neck is often due to an imbalance of the liver energy. To alleviate neck pain, take the same suggestions mentioned above and add the following:

- Lifting Qi Ball
- Separating Clouds
- Thump Pump on Neck

Press Small Intestine 3 for neck pain. First, move your neck into the position where you feel the most pain. Then press the point as hard as you can stand it. Relax and then repeat several times. You should feel almost immediate relief.

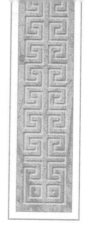

Bone Health

WHEN it comes to bone health, it is so important to think and act preventively, especially when you first begin to experience symptoms of menopause. Our bones have their own life cycle. Throughout our lives, they decline from the maximum bone mass reached during early adulthood to the slow bone loss characteristic of menopausal years. Osteoporosis occurs when normally dense bone tissue develops holes and spaces. The breakdown of the bone results in a net loss of the bone's mineral content and protein structure. If this process continues and the bones become weaker, more porous, and lighter, the chance of bone fracture increases.

Perimenopause is the time when calcium loss usually begins. Additional symptoms such as mood swings, menstrual irregularity, and hot flashes begin to occur in this period. Women can lose a tremendous amount of calcium over time, resulting in weakened bones. The amount of protein in the bone also contributes to flexibility and strength. Alternatively, excesses of many nutrients, such as too much calcium, and too much exercise can hasten bone loss.

In menopause, our bone mass may become even less concentrated as a result of inadequate nutrition, sedentary lifestyle, disturbed mental state, and ingestion of medications, alcohol, or other substances.

A regular program of movement and weight-bearing exercises stimulates the long bones of the legs and arms to maintain bone mass. The Twenty-Minute Workout provides qigong practice that can help you to maintain good posture and stronger bones, and, with its promotion of good balance, means you will be less likely to fall. Qigong provides you with a connection to the earth that energetically strengthens all 206 of your bones, helping you develop a strong sense of connection, support, structure, and safety in the world.

From a Chinese medical perspective, the kidneys govern and rule the "essence" of the bones and bone marrow. Strengthening the kidneys is the first line of defense against loss of bone density. Strengthening kidney qi allows bones to renew themselves more effectively. Practice the Healing Sound for Kidney and the entire Knitting Strong Bones set to improve bone health.

The endocrine system is also involved in maintaining bone strength. The parathyroid glands produce a hormone that helps to regulate calcium and phosphorus levels in your blood. The pituitary gland regulates the protein levels of the long bones. Osteoporosis can stem from various disorders of the thyroid, adrenals, and pancreas glands. For example, diabetes, a disorder of the pancreas gland, can cause osteoporosis because of its effect on vitamin D metabolism (vitamin D helps the body absorb calcium from the intestines). Therefore, practice the Energize Endocrine exercise of parathyroid, thyroid, adrenals, pancreas, and pituitary glands, sending love and attention to these precious hormone messengers.

ADDITIONAL TIPS FOR MAXIMIZING BONE STRENGTH ||

- If you eat meat, suck on the bones or drink a broth made from the bones for essential minerals. Meat, fish, and poultry strengthen the bones and tendons—of course organic meat is preferable because it is free of chemicals, antibiotics, and steroids.
- If you eat sardines or canned salmon and mackerel, buy the kind with bones in them to provide added calcium to your diet. Also choose to eat other small fish with bones.

- Eat foods naturally high in calcium such as dark green leafy vegetables, yogurt, hulled sesame seeds, tofu, soybeans, and broccoli. Ingest other mineral-rich foods for added bone nutrition from spring water and sea vegetables. Get adequate nonmeat protein, which is also an important component of strong bone structure and flexibility. This can be obtained from a combination of whole grains, beans, seeds, legumes, vegetables (especially yellow and orange vegetables and the cruciferous variety including cabbage, cauliflower, broccoli, and turnips), olive, flaxseed, sesame, and sunflower oils, and small amounts of animal protein and butter.

- Avoid drinking sodas because they can contain phosphoric acid, which leaches calcium from the bones and is a major contributing factor in the increase of osteoporosis.

- Limit your consumption of alcohol, refined sugar, and caffeine.

- Eat healthy, nutritious, organic, unrefined, and fresh foods. Eat well and nourish yourself with proper amounts of clean, healthy food throughout the menopause years. Make sure to eat plenty! This is essential for nourishing your qi and blood, which directly affects the health of your bones.

- Don't let yourself get too thin.

- Refrain from smoking, which drains calcium from your bones.

- Spend more of your time outdoors as sunshine provides vitamin D, which is essential for your bones to absorb calcium from the intestines.

- Spend more than four hours per day on your feet. A sedentary lifestyle weakens bones. Get up and move around as much as possible.

- Exercise in a balanced way and avoid exercise fanaticism. Gentle exercise is one of the best things you can do to prevent bone loss and to strengthen your bone mass in the process. The positive pressure we place on our bones during exercise actually attracts calcium to those bones, helping to build them. However, it's okay if you miss a day, or days, of exercise if something comes up—be gentle with yourself.

- Get a baseline bone density screening either before or during perimenopause. Fractures don't usually occur, if at all, until we are in our seventies and eighties.

The bones in your spine are some of the most important in your body. As we age, our vertebrae can begin to compress, causing us literally to shrink in stature. This pressure on our spinal column is bad for our internal organs. To rejuvenate our spine, it is essential to maintain good posture, and qigong is a natural way to do this.

For a straight spine, practice:

- Monkey Stretches Up and Down
- Fluffing White Clouds
- Swan Stretches Her Wings. While you do this exercise, stretching and squeezing your hand, imagine the spaces between your vertebrae opening and closing with each movement. Visualize yourself cleansing these spaces as if they were a dirty sponge being squeezed out in water.

A helpful combination of acupoints to direct energy to the bones includes:

- Kidney 3
- Gallbladder 34
- Spleen 6
- Small Intestine 3
- Gallbladder 41

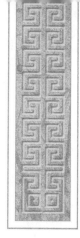

Breast Health

WHEN thinking of the health of our breasts in terms of Chinese medicine, we can look to the stomach meridian. The stomach meridian is so important because it runs straight up through the center of our breasts and affects the health of the whole breast.

Also of great importance to the breasts is the penetrating (*chong*) vessel. Drawing from a pool of 365 points located along the twelve meridians, this extraordinary vessel on the front torso spreads qi throughout the chest and connects our breasts to our uterus. Whatever happens to the breasts is connected to the qi of the uterus, and vice versa. Lumpy breasts are caused by stagnation within the penetrating vessel. The health of our nipples is governed by the way energy is flowing through our liver meridian. Furthermore, the liver and heart are pivotal organs when it comes to breast health because of their role in providing ample blood to the breasts, removing stagnation, and helping to process anger and sadness.

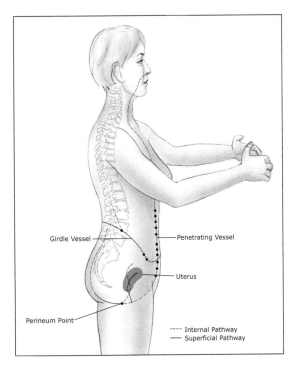

Girdle Vessel

Penetrating Vessel

Uterus

Perineum Point

---- Internal Pathway
— Superficial Pathway

● *Penetrating and Girdle Vessels*

❁ Sunburst Exercise *(1 minute)*

Stand with your feet parallel and a bit wider than your shoulders, knees slightly bent. As you stand with your palms facing your chest, imagine a steady stream of healing energy emanating from them. Bathe your breasts in this healing energy as you visualize healthy qi filling your breasts upon inhalation and stagnant qi leaving your breasts upon exhalation. Focus your attention to just behind your nipples and then allow the healing energy to emanate outward from your chest like a sunburst.

To expand this exercise, spread the healing qi by moving your hands first in a clockwise and then a counterclockwise direction. Send your breasts the positive energy they need to stay healthy for your entire life. Thank your breasts for providing nurturing energy and think about how much you appreciate this important, special part of your female body. Separating Clouds also promotes breast health. The motion of your arms in this exercise improves the energy flow from Large Intestine 15 located on the tip of each shoulder where the collarbone and the bone of the upper arm meet. Stimulate these points along with sending positive energy behind the center of each nipple, which balances the female hormonal system. These points are commonly used for prevention of breast cancer in China. Visualize the stimulation of these points when you practice Standing Like a Tree as well.

Acupressure points to create a free flow of energy and blood through the breasts include:

- Stomach 36
- Pericardium 6
- Liver 3

On an emotional level, it is essential for the health of your breasts that you release any anger or sadness that your body may be harboring. The liver meridian, which has to do with anger, and the heart meridian, which has to do with sadness, traverse in close proximity to the breasts. When these emotions are repressed, excessive, or unresolved, they can impair the function of the meridians associated with these organs and thus cause breast problems.

As little girls, many of us were taught never to show anger, that doing so was unladylike. But for our own health (not to mention the well-being of those who depend on us), it is crucial that we learn to release our emotions. We need to allow both the positive *and* so-called negative aspects of ourselves to coexist, to honor all of our feelings. Letting anger or sadness fester and linger increases our chance for problems in the breast area. So, please, express yourself! Saying what you feel when you feel it and in an appropriate manner will definitely make you feel better and you will have healthier breasts as a result.

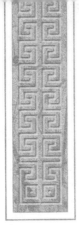

Breathing Difficulty

THE DEEP, slow, rhythmic breathing, which is an essential part of every exercise in the Twenty-Minute Workout, will naturally improve difficulties you may have with your breathing. The kind of deep breathing we do when we practice qigong brings a maximum amount of oxygen into our lungs and allows complete release of carbon monoxide. Because the lungs clean the air and regulate downward flow of qi, strengthening lung qi creates easier breathing and makes us feel more centered and grounded.

Concentrate on the following exercises to open the chest and to ease and clear your breathing:

- Brushing Wind.
- Swan Stretches Her Wings
- Fluffing White Clouds
- Woman Connects with Heaven and Earth

The health of your kidneys also affects breathing capacity because when you inhale, the kidneys "grab" qi from the lungs and thus promote and regulate inhalation. Practice the Kidney Rub for Life (page 103) as an essential component of your special qigong program for optimal breathing.

If you suffer from difficult breathing, add Beating Sky Drum to your normal workout. This exercise takes fifteen seconds to complete and breaks up congestion in the chest, alleviates coughs, and releases chest pain. Stand with your feet shoulder-width apart, parallel to each other with your knees slightly bent. Bend your arms up behind you to about the level of the bottom of your breasts. With loose fists, tap yourself vigorously on your back about an inch and a half from either side of your spine. Move your fists down your back, still tapping, to the level immediately behind your solar plexus, right below your rib cage.

Sometimes, breathing difficulty is simply caused by tightness in the muscles surrounding the rib cage. Releasing these muscles can increase lung capacity. Massage the spaces between your ribs on your chest and torso to release tension there and to improve breathing capacity.

Foods that are beneficial to the lungs include hot, spicy foods such as ginger and garlic and those white in color such as bananas, tofu, and rice. If you are suffering from a lung illness such as asthma, the following is a list of beneficial foods: figs, pumpkin, pears, honey, walnuts, carrots, kiwi, sunflower seeds, molasses, mustard greens, and sesame seeds. Molasses can be easily ingested by adding a tablespoon to a cup of boiled water to create a delicious drink that will nourish your lungs and boost your iron levels. One of my favorite dishes for strengthening the lungs is baked pears with honey and chopped walnuts sprinkled on top.

Shortness of breath can be due to a deficiency of heart and spleen energy. In addition to strengthening the qi of the lungs, the combination of the following acupressure points addresses heart and spleen as well as lungs:

- Conception Vessel 17
- Lung 1
- Conception Vessel 12
- Stomach 25

Another exercise, Breathing into Beautiful Belly, gets rid of stagnant air as it brings in fresh, clean air to oxygenate your blood. It massages your internal organs, detoxifies your body, and creates a sense of overall calm. Most important, this exercise will tone and strengthen your diaphragm, the part of your body that regulates the breath.

Lie down flat and place a lightweight object such as a tissue box on your belly. Breathe directly into your belly with your mouth closed, breathing in and out through your nostrils. Notice the object on your belly rise and fall. Breathe this way until it begins to feel natural. Take away the object and concentrate more deeply on your breathing.

Upon inhalation, notice your rib cage expanding. Visualize your diaphragm moving downward toward your feet, your belly expanding outward like inflating a balloon. Upon exhalation, notice your rib cage contract and move downward. As your belly contracts, visualize your diaphragm moving upward toward your head. This upward and downward motion of the diaphragm increases your lung capacity and massages your internal organs. It naturally forces the carbon dioxide out of your lungs so that you are ready to take in good, clean air upon inhalation.

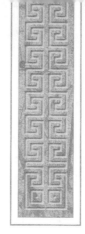

Coldness/Poor Circulation

POOR circulation is a common problem, especially as we grow older. However, you don't have to be older to experience lack of blood flow to your hands and feet. As women, we have a predominantly yin nature, so we often feel colder than men—yes, we are usually the ones with the cold tootsies in bed! But we can warm up and stay warmer permanently by balancing the yin and yang energy of our bodies through the qi- and blood-enhancing practice of qigong.

Qigong exercises for warming up the body include:

- Waking Up Qi Set
- Brushing Wind
- Thump Pump
- Lady Raises Lotus to the Temple
- Healing Sound for Heart
- Energize Endocrines for Hypothalamus and Pituitary

If you experience coldness, eliminate cold, raw foods and cold drinks from your diet. Eat mostly cooked, warm foods and drinks that are either room temperature or warm. Enjoy soups, cooked vegetables, baked or dry fruits, and smaller amounts of meat, fish, and poultry. These dietary guidelines are especially important in the winter months but should also be followed in warmer seasons because many people suffering from coldness feel cold in the summer months as well. The coldness is a sign that your blood is not properly nourishing your body. You need blood to nourish your tissues, prevent pain, and to keep all organs in good working order. Do as much as you can to increase body temperature on a regular basis!

Note: Chinese dietary principles teach that meat is medicine in small amounts, especially when a person is weak or deficient. Choose meats free from steroids, antibiotics, and other synthetic chemicals. Choose deep-sea fish such as red snapper or halibut over hatchery-grown fish such as salmon. Choose smaller fish over larger because they are lower on the food chain with less concentration of chemicals and other toxic substances.

Essential for warmth is a healthy spleen, which helps produce blood and nourishment for your system. It also controls your hands and feet, so when you're cold, deficient spleen yang may be the culprit.

Press acupressure points to warm your entire system:

- Triple Warmer 5 releases stagnant qi to open blood flow
- Stomach 36 strengthens flow of qi and blood
- Spleen 6 spreads liver qi, benefits kidneys and spleen, and builds blood especially when combined with Stomach 36

Cold hands and feet, a pale complexion, and an aversion to cold are caused internally by a deficiency of kidney yang in our bodies. As previously explained, yin relates to cold and yang relates to heat. When we are cold, this may mean there is a deficiency of kidney fire. Externally, this same pattern happens when you experience extremely cold exterior conditions such as frigid temperatures. In order to get warmer, we need to stoke that kidney fire. To do so:

avoid anything, anyplace, or anyone that makes you feel cold
don't overindulge in sex

sleep with socks to warm the Bubbling Well point

refrain from walking barefoot on cold floors

keep the lower back covered, especially in cold weather

avoid cold food and drinks, especially with ice or straight from the refrigerator

include some unrefined, unprocessed salty foods in your diet since salt nourishes the kidneys

drink ginger tea

use ginger compresses on your lower back or soak your feet in a ginger tea footbath

Make ginger tea by grating a quarter of an inch of fresh ginger into two cups of water. Bring to a boil and simmer gently for twenty minutes. To make a ginger compress, triple the water and ginger amount in the recipe for ginger tea. Use this ginger decoction in three ways to raise the yang energy of your body, which incidentally also wards off cold or flu. Either dip a cotton cloth in it, wring it out slightly, and place your back, wrap the cloth around both feet, or place the decoction (adding more hot water) in a big container and soak your feet.

To futher stoke your kidneys concentrate on:

- Kidney Rub for Life (page 103)
- Beautiful Woman Turns at Waist
- Monkey Stretches Up and Down

Do acupressure on:

- Kidney 3 to balance yin and yang energies of the kidneys
- Stomach 36 to strengthen weakness and deficiency

The liver governs the free flow of energy throughout the body. Therefore, coldness can also stem from liver problems, namely deficiency of blood (yin) of the liver and stagnation of liver qi. Put simply, the liver stores the blood. We know that a poor blood flow through the body leads to coldness. When the qi of the liver is not flowing properly, this stagnant qi won't move the blood. Anger, too, is an emotion associated with stagnant liver energy. If you are angry, you may be so tense that your blood won't flow properly and you feel cold, especially in your extremities. For better circulation, learn to express your anger in a positive way! Speak your mind, express your feelings, and avoid holding things in unless expressing them would be detrimental to yourself or others. Allow feelings to surface and, in addition to understanding where they come from, learn simply to accept them. After going through this process, you may not even have to verbalize your feelings to anyone. Writing in a journal helps release pent-up feelings, too.

To nourish your liver, incorporate sour foods such as pickles, lemons, vinegar, plums, or cranberries into your diet. Green foods such as dark green leafy vegetables and seaweeds are also helpful.

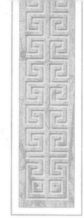

Constipation, Diarrhea, and Other Colon Issues

CONSTIPATION stems from excessive dryness combined with a deficiency of qi and blood. According to Chinese medicine, dryness prevents stools from being moistened. For women, constipation is often directly connected with the amount of blood flowing through our bodies, and a lack of blood leads to dryness. Plus, lack of energy, or deficient qi, hinders the ability to move stools through your system.

The organs mostly involved in constipation are the liver and kidneys. When we are constipated, these organs are yin deficient. Dryness of the stools also occurs when there is disharmony between the kidney and heart energies, or water and fire respectively. When there is too much heat and not enough fluid in your body, you may experience burning when you have a bowel movement. The key to becoming more regular is to balance the basic elements of fire and water. We do this by nourishing the yin of the kidneys, giving them the ability to produce enough water to balance the fire element. We soothe the fire of liver and heart so it doesn't burn or scorch bodily fluids. Avoid barbecued or fried foods also, as these can cause excessive heat in the body.

Do the following to strengthen kidneys and soothe fire within the liver and heart:

- Rag Doll Twist
- Spinning Wheel
- Back Swinging Monkey
- Healing Sounds for Kidneys, Liver, and Heart

To alleviate constipation, the kidneys need to produce more water, but this does not simply mean you should drink more water. Yes, it is important to drink enough water, but too much can stress your kidneys. Instead of thinking only about drinking eight glasses a day, listen to your individual body needs to keep yourself hydrated. Drink high-quality water, herbal teas, vegetable and fruit juices, soy and rice milk or other healthy liquids to quench your thirst.

The goal is to balance yin and yang energies, or water and fire inside your body, to create a proper balance of bodily organ functions and fluids. To do this through qigong practice:

- Standing Like a Tree
- Walking Like a Turtle
- Bone Washing
- Lady Raises Lotus to the Temple
- Feeling Qi performed in Horse Stance

HEALTHY ELIMINATION SUGGESTIONS

Colon and intestinal health is essential for good health. Having a complete bowel movement once or twice a day is important for releasing toxins from your system. This keeps your colon and intestines free from buildup of old residue, which can get stuck in the intestinal crevices and lead to colon disease.

To encourage your body to produce a complete, regular bowel movement, set aside the same time(s) every day to relieve yourself. Creating a rhythm within your elimination system promotes bowel regularity. You may do best after getting out of bed, after a warm morning drink, or after eating breakfast. If the afternoon or evening works better for you, so be it. Creating a consistent time is most important for establishing a reliable elimination cycle. Go to the bathroom when you get the urge rather than holding it in. Place your feet on a bench or footstool about a foot off the ground while on the toilet to help promote smooth elimination.

As anyone who suffers from constipation knows, it's almost impossible to have a bowel movement when you don't relax. Reading in the bathroom can help as movement of the eyes while reading helps evacuation, but don't sit on the toilet too long, since this can lead to hemorrhoids. Rubbing the upper *dantian* point just above and between your eyes for fifteen to thirty seconds also relaxes the bowels and allows elimination to occur more swiftly, gently, and completely. The following two exercises also relieve constipation:

Relaxing Bowels Exercise:

Before sitting down, take a mouthful of water but don't swallow it. Squat down with your knees bent and your feet shoulder-width apart. Lift up your heels, placing most of your weight on your toes. Extend your arms and fists straight out in front of you at shoulder height. Swallow in three separate "swallows." Swallow the first two with a hard gulp and the third with a natural, gentle motion. This should help to create the urge to eliminate your bowels immediately. This entire process takes twenty seconds.

Great Eliminator Exercise *(30 seconds to 1 minute or more)*

You can also give yourself a qigong massage of your abdomen without ever touching your belly. This is best done while on the toilet, as you will be right there ready to release or push out the contents of your colon. If you really concentrate your mind on what you are doing and believe, it works like a charm. The purpose of this exercise is obviously to eliminate your bowels, but also to strengthen your intestines. This is similar to Set 4, in which you send love and attention to your endocrine glands. With the abdomen "massage," you can see actual physical results right away. One of the most crucial aspects of this exercise is to hone your intention. Make certain that your mind's eye goes inside the intestines so you "see" the waste moving through them. The

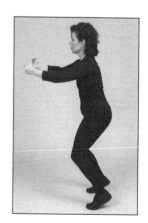
● *Relaxing Bowels Exercise*

more you practice this exercise, the better it works. When your intent is clear, your qi will follow its path. When the qi arrives in your intestines, the blockage will resolve and the stools will move.

First, place your palms facing your abdomen with fingertips pointed toward each other. Without touching your abdomen, send qi into your intestines and colon. Follow the path of the intestines with the movement of your hands. Begin on the bottom right side of your abdomen, up the ascending colon, to the bottom of the rib cage, then across your abdomen, across the transverse colon to the bottom of the left rib cage (see figure on page 98). Now move your hands down the left side of your abdomen, along the descending colon. Follow this path to relieve constipation. Imagine that your fingers are nudging the contents of your intestines and colon along and out of your body. Use a wavelike motion, moving your fingers in small circles as you inch them along. As you sit on the toilet, press Large Intestine 4 on your right hand. This point itself is known as the Great Eliminator and it does just that!

Enhance the effectiveness of any of these methods by drinking a glass of water mixed with the juice of half of a lemon before starting. If the constipation is due to medication, accept that it may be more difficult to budge. If you don't get results right away, repeat these techniques immediately or a little later. Remain patient in this process and hope for the best.

DIARRHEA AND IRRITABLE BOWEL SYNDROME

Diarrhea is a condition associated with excessive dampness of the spleen. The spleen governs transformation and transportation of food in your system. When the spleen's transformation function is impaired, we experience either diarrhea or constipation. Irritable bowel syndrome (IBS) can be due to either kidney deficiency leading to dryness or spleen deficiency leading to dampness, or both. The emotions, too, have a direct effect on the presence of diarrhea and IBS. Any of the exercises in the Twenty-Minute Workout are excellent in calming the emotions, but Swans Stretches Her Wings specifically strengthens the spleen energy, alleviating both diarrhea and IBS-related symptoms.

If you have diarrhea, practice the Great Eliminator exercise described above for constipation, but reverse the direction, and thus the path of qi. Begin on your left side and move up the descending colon with a gentle circular motion that promotes the reabsorption of water into your intestines. Continue with this gentle, soothing circular motion across the transverse colon and down the ascending colon to help create well-formed stools. As you do this exercise, visualize your stool becoming formed and dry. Acupressure on Stomach 44 and Spleen 9 helps with this process as well.

In Chinese medicine, diarrhea and constipation are opposite sides of the same coin, one condition caused by dampness, the other by dryness. If you have both problems, perform the massage in both directions. If you wish to maintain the general health of your colon, simply flutter your fingers and make circular movements, sending good healthy qi and appreciation into this wonderful organ that helps eliminate poisons and unwanted substances from your body.

Other Acupressure points:

- Large Intestine 11 removes heat and therefore excessive dryness from the intestines
- Stomach 25 stimulates blood and qi flow and directly treats the bowels
- Spleen 4 for intestines that are "hard like a drum"
- Gallbladder 34 for habitual constipation

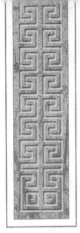

Depression and Irritability

DEPRESSION and irritability are all too common for women, especially in the years after our periods stop. In many cases, just doing your Twenty-Minute Workout will help you find greater joy and peace of mind. Depression is a complex issue, with many organs involved. At base, most depression and irritability for women stems from accumulation of phlegm and stagnation of liver qi. In Chinese medicine, we alleviate depression and irritability by clearing up phlegm, relaxing the liver energy, and reducing or eliminating the stagnation of qi.

The liver is responsible for creating ample and free flow of qi and blood in the body. If the liver is not functioning properly, it impedes the digestive function. When this happens, a woman cannot properly absorb nutrition and thus can't nourish her body with essential nutrients for life. The undigested food turns into excessive phlegm.

The liver is quite temperamental and easily affected, especially by anger. Excessive anger and stress can severely impair the liver's ability to create free flow of energy and blood through the body. Anger makes the qi rebellious, causing it to flow upward. This is that irritable feeling that makes us fly off of the handle. When the liver is not creating a free flow of energy through the body, one is suffering from constrained liver qi. When this constraint goes on for an extended period of time, the qi in the liver becomes stagnant. This is when we become depressed.

Excessive sitting also makes stagnation of liver qi worse because blood in our arms and legs goes to the liver to be stored. During exercise, blood is pumped out of the liver, reducing any qi that has become stuck in the system. Qigong, self-acupressure, and a balanced diet smooth and redirect liver qi to flow freely.

Foods that, when used to excess, irritate the liver include: alcohol, coffee, red meat, and greasy, fatty, fried, barbecued, spicy, hot, acrid, and pungent dishes. Preservatives, chemicals, coloring agents, artificial flavors, hard-to-digest foods, too much food, and prescription or over-the-counter drugs make the liver work extra hard in its detoxification process.

The combination of prolonged liver qi stagnation, excessive stress, and improper diet can turn the stagnation into heat and even fire. This form of excessive heat or fire in the liver can be aggravated by a phenomenon called raging minister fire, a kind of flare-up that itself is ignited by emotional distress, lots of anger, frustration, and feelings of hatred. Raging minister fire is localized at *mingmen*, the Life Gate Fire point.

When minister fire is quiet, tranquil, and balanced, it nourishes the water of the body rather than burning it up. But when excessive emotions are present, this fire becomes agitated and burns up the vital substances of the body. Thus, the combination of liver fire and minister fire consuming the vital fluids in your body can lead to a devastating heat condition. Such an imbalance also causes depression and irritability in addition to a host of gynecological problems. If you are always furious, hateful, constantly yelling, angry, tense, have severely dry skin and a parched mouth, and most of all feel totally "burned out" you may have raging minister fire.

Patients are often amazed to find a question on my intake form about "plum pit throat," a symptom indicative of liver stagnation. Though many have experienced the sensation that something is stuck in their throat, few were ever questioned by a health care provider about it. Constantly clearing your throat or coughing to remove the "pit" without success means you probably have plum pit throat. It is a sensation similar to that feeling you get when you are beginning to cry and stop yourself. This symptom is indicative of a liver energy imbalance that stems from unprocessed, stuck emotions such as sadness or anger.

If you think you might have plum pit throat, arrange to have an emotional release in a secluded, private place. Scream and cry to release your pent-up rage as often as you deem necessary.

On your path to becoming ageless, it is important that you express your anger to others clearly, lovingly, and in the right times. If not treated, stagnation of liver qi causes the mind to become obstructed. In advanced stages, this condition can even lead to mental disturbance of the kind we see when women have severe postpartum depression.

Practice Spinning Wheel to facilitate smooth flow of liver qi and release of qi stagnation. Woman Connects with Heaven and Earth also lifts feelings of depression.

Practice Beautiful Woman Turns at Hips to stimulate the flow of energy in the girdle vessel (see illustration page 174) that circles the waist. This meridian is extremely important in women's physiology because it promotes the free and smooth flow of liver qi. Beautiful Woman Turns at Hips can be very helpful in preventing stagnation or a fire condition in the liver.

According to the five elements, the kidneys nourish the liver and control the heart. Deficiency of the kidney energy and lack of harmony between the kidneys and the heart also affects one's mood. Calming your mind and spirit is essential when balancing the heart energy, as the heart houses the mind and nourishes the spirit. The lungs, too, are involved in depression. The governing emotion of the lungs is grief. When a woman experiences a death in the family, a divorce, or loses a beloved friend or pet, she may cover up her feelings and not express her grief completely. When this happens, the grief is unresolved and injures the lungs, leading to depression and sadness. Crying is a good way of releasing sad, grieving energy held within the lungs. The spleen plays a role in our mood, too. When there is deficiency within the spleen, there is excess dampness, which drowns the body in water and constrains the mind. This prevents us from making decisions and keeps us trapped thinking the same stale thoughts, leading to depression and frustration.

In summary, the liver, kidneys, heart, lungs, and spleen are intricately connected with symptoms of depression and irritability. Remember, it's all connected in Chinese medicine.

The Five Healing Sounds, which bolster the health of all these organs, can be very beneficial in relieving feelings of depression and irritability. This exercise helps reduce stress and promotes relaxation. It works with the mind as well as the body. When doing these healing sounds for all five of the organs, add to your practice an inner smile. As you are performing this set, think of happy times in your life. Make sure that you have a beautiful, warm, relaxed smile on your face and imagine that you are bestowing that sweet smile on your internal organs, creating balance and the healing of your emotional state. Take your time visualizing your loving and joyful energy flowing within as you practice this set.

There is a Chinese saying, "Laughter can take away ten years of aging." And there is a Western saying that, "Every time you cry, you add another day to your life." If you want to live a long and healthy life, release your tears and laugh a lot. Balance is also important, however. Crying too much injures the lungs, stomach, and spleen and excessive laughing is indicative of heart fire.

Also for mental depression and agitation, give yourself acupressure on:

- Pericardium 6 to calm your emotions
- Spleen 4 to shift your emotional state
- Liver 3 to create free flow of qi and blood
- Conception Vessel 17 to stimulate the endorphins and reduce melancholy

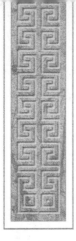

Digestive Problems

CHINESE medicine views the transformation and transportation of food as governed by the spleen. According to the flow of energy in the law of the five elements, the liver controls the spleen and the stomach (the spleen's sister organ). Therefore, digestion is commonly affected by liver energy. The liver regulates stomach qi, is responsible for directing it downward, and is associated with upsetting emotions. This is why, whenever you are upset about something, your stomach gets upset, too. Avoid eating when you are extremely upset, angry, or anxious.

Problems with the digestion occur when there is a stagnation of qi related to the liver and an accumulation of phlegm related to the spleen. This becomes a vicious cycle. Phlegm and stagnation come from poor digestion, but poor digestion in turn causes excess phlegm and stagnation.

The kidneys' job is to nourish the liver and warm the spleen, so the kidneys, too, are key to healthy digestion.

Heartburn comes from excessive heat in the stomach due to general overeating. That hot, burning sensation can occur even when you eat small amounts of certain foods or when your stomach is too empty. This leads to disharmony of the heart and liver. Heartburn also comes from a deficiency of yin (water) of the liver and kidneys. This leads to a flaring of fire in the digestive region. Whether your digestive problems are caused by too much fire or by too much water, they can be quickly helped by doing the exercises suggested below.

- Fluffing White Clouds and Feeling Qi strengthen the stomach and spleen energy and thereby promote healthy digestion.
- Practice Healing Sounds for Spleen, Liver, and Heart thirty-six times each.
- Swan Stretches Her Wings strengthens digestion and elimination and adjusts and regulates the function of the stomach, spleen, heart, and liver.
- Energize Endocrines for Pancreas to create digestive enzymes to metabolize foods, produce insulin, and regulate blood sugar.
- Woman Connects with Heaven and Earth strengthens the spleen, kidney, and liver energies and therefore helps promote transportation and transformation of food in the body.
- Horse Stance strengthens digestion and elimination.

When there is a deficiency in your digestive function, follow these helpful tips:

- Eat only cooked foods. The heat from the cooking aids your digestion by breaking down the food somewhat before it reaches your belly.
- Eat bland foods and avoid any additives such as artificial colors. Stay away from hot and spicy, fried, or processed food.
- Take your time. Always chew your food as many times as possible prior to swallowing. Before eating, stop to notice and appreciate the food in front of you.
- If you are having digestive poblems, remember this at your daily meals: when you eat, eat! Make sure you're sitting down, concentrate on your food, try not to read, avoid excessive talking, and don't drink fluids while eating since it interferes with the digestive process.
- Brown rice, millet, oats, barley, sweet rice, carrots, papaya, winter squash, honey, and sweet yellow or orange foods such as yams and sweet potatoes nourish the spleen and promote healthy digestion.

■ Singing is said to be healing for the spleen as well (but don't sing while you eat!).

On an emotional level, problems with digestion often arise when we do not treat ourselves with the respect we deserve, when we do not honor our "contract" with ourselves. What does this mean? Simply put, it is the concept that we are on earth for unique reasons, to live the life only we can live. If we neglect our duty to ourselves or our calling, if we allow our relationships with others to determine our lives, we often feel in our gut that something is wrong. We may develop problems in our digestive organs. In order to remedy this, we must make a commitment within ourselves to honor and live out our personal contracts. Only then are we able to depend on ourselves, doing and saying only those things that are truly right for us. By being true to ourselves, we are able to have smooth, honest, loving relationships with others, and to "digest" what the world offers us in a healthy way.

The Fire Belly exercise (45 seconds to 1 minute) is a useful addition for strengthening digestion. Lie down in a comfortable position. Place a light object such as a tissue box on your abdomen and watch it rise on the inhalation and fall on the exhalation. Then remove the object and repeat the same exercise with your hands resting gently on your abdomen. Imagine that your abdomen is a balloon filling with air on the inhalation and deflating upon exhalation, just as you did in Breathing into Beautiful Belly. Next, with your hands still on your abdomen, place your fingertips on your navel and begin rubbing clockwise. Start with smaller circles and progress to larger and larger circles. At the same time, increase the speed of your massage until you feel warmth emanating from your belly. This exercise stokes your digestive fire and at the same time stimulates the area the Chinese refer to as the stove.

Acupressure to strengthen the stove includes pressing the following points:

■ Conception Vessel 12 regulates stomach qi
■ Stomach 36 creates order of the spleen and stomach
■ Liver 9 promotes the free flow of energy in the liver meridian
■ Spleen 9 transforms stagnation of dampness

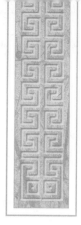

Dizziness

DIZZINESS occurs when we do not have enough blood nourishing our head, when there is fire raging in our body, or when we have a deficiency of vital energy. According to Chinese medicine, dizziness occurs when: 1) the kidneys are not sparking and nourishing the energy and water of the body, and 2) the liver is not promoting the free flow of energy and blood, not storing enough blood, and/or creating excessive heat in the system, and 3) the heart is not sending enough blood circulating through the system.

Essentially, this knot of problems leaves those suffering from dizziness without sufficient quality water or blood. When this continues over an extended period of time, it turns into an excessive heat pattern. In this case, you will have symptoms such as red cheeks, night sweating, dryness, mental restlessness, irritability, dry throat, and hot flashes. It can be difficult to move from one place to another when you feel so dizzy, but the following exercises will help.

You may need to practice the first six of the following exercises in a seated position and then get up and do the walking exercise slowly, with tiny steps.

Always move slowly as you shift from sitting to standing, and into a walking position. You will soon find that when your qi is flowing better, so will your blood, and the dizziness will be resolved (this happens because qi moves blood). Practice:

- Shaking the Tree to release qi and blood blockages (page 165)
- Feeling Qi to build your qi
- Fluffing White Clouds to nourish your blood
- Healing Sound for Liver thirty-six times to detoxify and release heat from your liver
- Beating the Heavenly Drum to promote alertness and blood circulation to the head
- Kidney Rub for Life (page 103) to spark the kidneys, the root of the energy for all of your organs
- Walking Like a Turtle to harmonize your yin and yang energies

In order to relieve dizziness, practice self-acupressure on the following points:

- Governing Vessel 26, a revival point
- Spleen 6 to nourish your blood
- Stomach 36 together with Spleen 6 to nourish and strengthen the blood

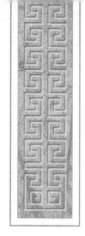

Dryness

WHETHER of the face, hair, eyes, nose, mouth, vagina, or clitoris, dryness in the body comes internally from deficiency of blood due to lack of fluids and/or excess heat. Externally, it stems from environmental elements. Dryness is a common problem for women because blood is such a precious commodity for us, especially as we get older. To combat dryness, we need to stay relaxed emotionally, drink enough but not too much water and other fluids, eat healthy foods that nourish blood, avoid extreme hot or dry climates (indoor and out), and do exercises that move blood. More specifically, it is essential to nourish the blood of the liver because this is what moistens the skin. If liver blood becomes deficient, the skin is dry and even itchy. This happens frequently during menopause and can be especially the case for you if you have always had light or irregular periods. Dry, itchy skin is also common for menopausal women who have always been cold and for women with pale complexions; both symptoms are indicative of blood deficiency.

For dryness practice:

- Swan Stretches Her Wings
- Phoenix Eats Its Ashes
- Healing Sound for Liver
- Rag Doll Twist

The Conception Vessel that runs up the front and the Governing Vessel that runs down the back center of the body are both crucial to maintaining a healthy balance of blood, qi, water and fire, or yin and yang in our bodies. When yin and yang are out of balance, it can lead to dryness (as well as a host of other problems). One way to rectify dryness is to move energy up the back and down the front of your body through the Microcosmic Orbit. The Microcosmic Orbit ensures a proper balance of elements within your body so your tissues maintain a proper amount of fluid.

MICROCOSMIC ORBIT

Stand or sit up straight, whether on a pillow on the floor or on a chair. Rest your hands on your *dantian* and close your eyes halfway. Empty your mind, create calmness within, and concentrate on your slow deep, and rhythmical breaths. Move your attention downward, and concentrate on the perineum point. Inhale and with your mind's eye follow the governing vessel up through the midline of your back to the crown of your head. As you exhale, follow the conception vessel downward through the front center of your body back to the *dantian* where the qi is stored. These two vessels are not connected at the top, but you can create a connection by placing your tongue gently on the roof of your mouth throughout the visualization.

The touch of your tongue on the roof of your mouth is referred to as building the bridge. It is as if you are flipping an electrical switch that completes the electrical circuit between the governing and conception vessels. Placing the tongue too hard, too tight, or too far back on the roof of your mouth can cause stagnation of qi flow within these vessels. If your tongue is placed too far forward and touches your teeth, it can lead to an incomplete connection and even make you feel so tired you want to sleep. With a good connection, saliva will appear in the mouth. Swallow this saliva to keep the throat moistened as you perform the Microcosmic Orbit. As you visualize the movement of energy upward, then downward, do so gently and with focused intent. You may feel the flow of energy within your body as a tingling sensation. Practice this exercise for three rounds around the orbit. It is fine to do fifteen to twenty repetitions at a time.

WRINKLES

Chinese medicine views wrinkles as dryness and considers them a deficient blood issue. When we go out and face the world, it is important that we feel good about how we look. Being content with your looks is an essential component of good mental and physical health. In addition to the suggestions above for dryness, enlivening the face through self-acupressure brings additional blood and qi to this region and helps eliminate wrinkles. The self-acupressure points for preventing and reducing wrinkles are:

- Stomach 3 for your cheeks
- Gallbladder 14 for your eyes and forehead
- Stomach 4 for your smile lines
- Conception Vessel 24 for your chin and neck
- Governing Vessel 26 for above your lip
- Stomach 6 for jowels
- *Yintang* for brow or frown line
- *Taiyang* for crowsfeet

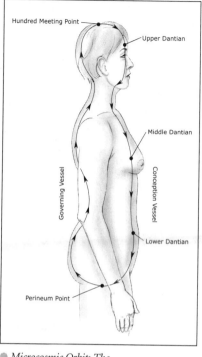

● *Microcosmic Orbit: The circular pathway designated with arrows in an internal pathway running from the* dantian *up the back centerline (Governing Vessel) to the Hundred Meeting point and then down the front centerline (Conception Vessel) to the perineum point.*

Combine the pressing of these points with gentle massage on your face and scalp followed by gentle tapping with your fingertips. Make sure not to miss your neck.

Another natural favorite for soft, smooth skin is to apply a facial mask of raw honey all over your face and neck. As the honey sticks to your fingers, tap your face gently. It feels fabulous! Leave the honey on for five to ten minutes, wash off with moderately hot water, and then spritz your face with mineral water. Let your skin dry naturally and then place a thin layer of natural moisturizer on your face and neck.

Healthy lung and spleen qi also helps you look your best. The lungs nourish the skin so it is essential for wrinkle-free skin that your lung energy be strong and balanced. Brushing Wind will help. The spleen energy is also important for reducing wrinkles and cellulite. This is due to the spleen's role in processing foods and making blood in the body. In addition to taking time with your food, eat clean and nutritious foods, and also practice Swan Stretches Her Wings for your spleen qi.

Foods that nourish the lungs include plums, persimmons, almonds, honey, and onions. Nourishing your spleen through food is discussed in the section on digestion (page 192).

WATER RETENTION

While dryness is caused by not enough blood, leading to yin deficiency, excess water or dampness within the body is due to not enough qi, leading to yang deficiency. When you retain water, it is because there is not enough fire in the body to process excess water, so the water stagnates in the system. This leads to what the Chinese call excess dampness, which could also be caused by extreme damp weather or living conditions.

When you have water retention, it means you are kidney or spleen yang deficient. When you have kidney yang deficiency, you may also be pale, swollen, and averse to cold. You may have cold limbs, lack energy, have low back soreness and clear, excess, or scant urine. If you have spleen yang deficiency, you may feel heavy, especially in the head and limbs. Or you may have trouble losing weight, be extremely tired, or experience secretions such as thick matter coming from your eyes. The best way to lessen this problem is by practicing the Thump Pump, mini yin massage, and the entire Waking Up Qi set to help move water through the body. Be patient because dampness can be stubborn. Do self-acupressure on the following points:

- Spleen 9 to transform dampness
- Large Intestine 4 to eliminate excess water
- Kidney 3 to benefit the kidneys

Avoid ingesting cold, raw food. Such foods aggravate dampness. When our spleen energy is already weak, raw foods are more difficult to digest. Be kind to your spleen and feed yourself only cooked or dried foods. Drink one to two cups of ginger tea (page 181) per day to help rid your body of excess dampness.

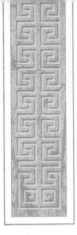

Eyesight Problems

LIVER energy nourishes your eyes, so the free flow of energy within your liver meridian is essential for healthy eyesight. Conversely, too much "looking," whether from many hours at the computer, watching television, or even reading, can injure our liver energy. In addition, deficiency of the kidneys and lack of harmony between the kidneys and heart can lead to blurred vision. Practice qigong exercises that nourish the blood of the liver, promote free flow of energy in the liver meridian, strengthen kidney energy, and calm the mind.

For eye and vision health:

- Spinning Wheel
- Beating the Heavenly Drum
- Healing Sounds for Liver, Heart, and Kidney
- A gentle mini yin massage around your eyes, face, scalp, and neck increases circulation

Many people begin wearing glasses too soon. There are other ways to strengthen your vision without the use of glasses. You may have noticed that the more you wear glasses, the worse your eyes get. See if you are able to use your glasses only during periods of extensive reading or while driving for extra support or safety. Attempt to get away with not using them at other times. Doing the qigong exercise for your eyes can help to strengthen them naturally.

The lycii berry, a little, red dried fruit available in Asian markets, is considered great medicine for eyes (these are different than the similarly named lychee). Buy a bag of lycii berries, store them in a sealed jar, and snack on a small handful once a day. Lycii berries are sweet yet sour, and best of all great for eyes and blood. Eating broccoli is also reputed to brighten eyes.

Two extraordinary meridians, the yin and yang heel vessels (*yin qiao* and *yang qiao*), both flow from the heels to the eyes. The yin heel vessel carries yin energy to the eyes and the yang heel vessel carries yang energy to the eyes. The yin heel vessel is traditionally used to treat eye diseases by pressing the acupoint Kidney 6. The yang heel vessel can be treated by pressing Urinary Bladder 62. You can also do acupressure on the points located around the eyes: Gallbladder 14 above the eyes, *taiyang* at your temples, and Stomach 3 on your cheeks. Added to Gallbladder 41 and Liver 3 on the top of the feet, you have an effective, easy treatment for vision problems.

❀ Healing Eyes Exercise *(3 minutes, 30 seconds)*

For best effect, do this combination of eye exercises on a daily basis. You can do them while walking the dog, waiting in traffic, sitting at your desk, before beginning your Twenty-Minute Workout, or at any other time that suits your needs. They can be done sitting, standing, or lying down.

Open your eyes as wide as you can, then shut them as tight as you can. Repeat this six times (10 seconds).

Facing straight ahead and with your eyes open, circle your eyes twelve times clockwise and twelve times counterclockwise (40 seconds). Next, looking as far out into the distance as you can, focus your eyes and then bring them down and focus at a point on the ground in front of you. Repeat this twelve times (1 minute). Next, look as far as you can to your right and then as far as you can to your left side, moving just your eyes but not your head. Repeat this a total of twelve times—six times to the right and six times to the left (30 seconds).

Finally, with your head facing forward and again without moving it up or down, look up and down with your eyes twelve times (30 seconds). To conclude this eye exercise, rub your palms together until they are very warm and place your hands over your eyes. With your palms over your eyes, gently massage around your eyes in small circles with pressure coming from your entire hand at once. Place your hands with the palms sides toward you over your entire face and take three deep breaths into your *dantian* (30 seconds). This completes your eye-strengthening qigong exercise.

Note: You may do any of these exercises up to thirty-six times if you wish.

If you are having trouble with your vision, don't forget to take stock on an emotional level. Is there something you need to "see" more clearly in your life? Give yourself time and space for precious insights to surface.

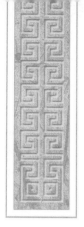

Fatigue/Weakness of Legs

FATIGUE can be due to a deficiency of the yang (fire) of the kidneys. This means that the spark of energy has waned in your body and you no longer have that get-up-and-go feeling. In addition to suffering fatigue and weakness in your legs, you might feel insecure, fearful, and find yourself complaining to others.

The Kidney Rub for Life (page 103) strengthens kidney yang, Beautiful Woman Turns at Waist boosts kidney qi, and practicing the Healing Sound for Kidneys detoxifies the kidneys.

While practicing your Twenty-Minute Workout, lift the corners of your mouth. This keeps your kidneys healthy and retards the aging process. Also, to preserve kidney energy, avoid excessive sex. Place a ginger compress on your lower back or soak your feet in a big pot of hot ginger water to strengthen your kidney energy (see ginger recipe, page 181).

The kidneys are instrumental along with the spleen in causing fatigue and weakness of the legs. The kidney sparks energy, providing you with get-up-

and-go. The spleen nourishes the muscles. The heart and liver provide adequate blood needed for strong legs.

Remember that blood is the mother of qi, but qi is the commander of blood, telling it where and how to move throughout the body. Without blood, qi has no substance, and vice versa. Without proper qi from the kidneys, blood from the heart and liver, and the spleen's nourishment of the muscles, our legs will not be able to get us where we need to go.

Do acupressure on the following points to move blood, strengthen qi, and thus counteract fatigue:

- Stomach 36 combined with Spleen 6
- Large Intestine 4
- Kidney 3
- Pericardium 6
- Liver 9

To eliminate weakness in the legs, practice Phoenix Eats Its Ashes and Tigress Crouches Down. The eight Standing Like a Tree postures and Walking Like a Turtle exercises promote strength of the legs and good balance as well. The Horse Stance (page 11) is another sure way to strengthen your legs. You can remain in it from three to ten minutes. (I used to practice Horse Stance for an hour a day, a typical duration when training in martial arts.)

Press the following acupoints to eliminate leg weakness:

- Gallbladder 41 strengthens the girdle vessel surrounding the hips (see illustration on page 156).
- Gallbladder 34 opens up flow of qi in the legs, strengthens tendons, ligaments, and bones, and helps with problems of the lower extremities.

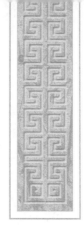

Hair Loss/Growth

HAIR loss on the head can be extremely common when hormones change, especially during pregnancy or after menopause. In order to treat this problem, we need to attend to our kidney energy because the kidneys nourish the hair on the head. Hair loss is also often due to excessive stress, which wreaks havoc on kidney energy. For this and for many other reasons, you must learn to modify the levels of stress in your life. Remember, you have options. Saying no when things get too much for you is the first line of defense against stress. To strengthen your kidney qi, practice:

- The Kidney Rub for Life (page 103)
- Healing Sound for Kidneys thirty-six times
- During the Energize Endocrines exercise, give extra love and appreciation to your adrenal glands since the adrenals and the kidneys are one and the same.

The kidneys can also be nourished with aduki beans, a little red bean with a black or white dot on them found in health food stores or Asian markets.

Prerinse then soak the beans overnight in water, remove beans, and drink one cup of the bean water with a dash of soy sauce in the water per day. Due to the salty taste, it will go directly to the kidneys. You can also eat the cooked beans. They are tasty with brown rice and hiziki seaweed or just lightly seasoned as a side dish. For strengthening your kidney energy, eat warm rather than cold foods and drinks, as the kidneys hate cold. Black beans, pine nuts, walnuts, plums, chicken, fish, and lamb are also effective food remedies for strengthening the kidneys.

The following are additions to the recommendations already listed on page 103 to protect the yin and yang aspects of your kidneys. Be careful not to sit on cold surfaces and make sure the rooms where you live and work are warm enough. Be conservative when it comes to sex because too much sex drains the energy from your kidneys. How much is too much depends on the individual. I would say once or twice a week is moderate for most women, every day or twice a day is excessive. Some women refrain from having an orgasm so they can recirculate their kidney essence (jing). This can be especially helpful while going through a healing process. We need to guard our precious kidney essence because we only last as long as it does.

To prevent hair loss, practice a daily qi scalp massage (30 seconds to 1 minute). Massage your scalp with your fingertips using small circles, starting at the front of the hairline and working your way back until you reach the nape of your neck. Keep contact the entire time, barely allowing your fingers to leave your scalp. Repeat this massage three to six times. Use a firm yet comfortable pressure. Some days you'll be able to press more deeply than others. If your scalp feels sensitive, be gentle. When you stimulate the acupressure points they often feel sensitive. This massage will increase blood circulation in the scalp and give you healthier hair.

After completing the qi scalp massage, take your fingertips and gently brush them through your hair, then softly tap your scalp; massage and brush from front to back (30 seconds). This qi massage stimulates all of the acupoints located on your head.

If you are experiencing growth of facial hair, another common problem as we age, attend to your penetrating vessel. Also called the Sea of Blood, this meridian influences the supply and proper movement of blood in the body. It also nourishes qi, and is related to body hair. If you have problems with facial hair, you can create an ample amount of qi and blood to properly moisten the skin by doing acupressure on the following penetrating vessel points:

- Spleen 4
- Pericardium 6

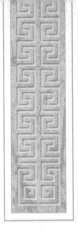

Headaches

FOR WOMEN, the most common cause of headaches is a deficiency of blood combined with what is called deranged qi due to excessive worry. Quite simply, this combination means that when we worry, not enough blood comes into the head. Women who have this type of headache usually feel cold and have pale complexions. They are also unable to relax. This type of headache is due to deficiency of liver blood.

Headaches are valuable warning signs saying that something is awry. Listen to the signs provided by the body and find ways through qigong to balance and heal yourself. Qigong treats root causes rather than just eliminating the symptom, known as the branch.

Women who suffer headaches need to learn how to relax. Holding a constant level of tension in the body restricts our qi flow, constraining the flow of blood and leading to awful headaches. During menopausal years, headaches can become worse as we naturally become more blood deficient. Combined with the hormonal changes, we are left headachy and thus more irritable. And keep in mind that the emotion of liver is anger. All combined, this leads to a vicious cycle of pain, anger, and unhappiness.

Exercise is a wonderful way to move the blood and qi and can be very helpful for alleviating headaches. Qigong is an excellent option because it is done to strengthen the body and calm the mind. Concentrate on the following exercises already in your Twenty-Minute Workout:

- Lady Raises Lotus to the Temple
- Lifting Qi Ball
- Spinning Wheel

When deficiency of liver blood turns into heat that rises up in the body, it can cause throbbing headaches at the top or sides of the head. This is often accompanied by blurred vision. This is extremely common for women, especially around their periods or during menopause. It is essential to eat foods that are nourishing to the blood, such as seaweed or lean red meat. Sour foods should be avoided as they cause more pain by disrupting the liver. These include foods such as oranges, grapefruits, vinegar, pickles, and yogurt.

Other common causes of headaches are sinus infections and allergies. These types of headaches are mainly due to weak qi in the lungs, not nourishing the nose adequately. They can also result from deficiency in the spleen, which doesn't process food properly or produce enough blood. If you experience headaches as a result of allergies or sinus infections, practice:

- Qi scalp massage (see page 208)
- Swan Stretches Her Wings to strengthen the spleen energy
- Brushing Wind to strengthen the lung energy
- Qigong massage on the abdomen to eliminate mucus via the intestines (page 185)

Drink one or two cups of ginger tea (recipe on page 181) per day to cut through and break down mucus. Eat prunes or flax seeds (delicious added to oatmeal) to promote increased bowel elimination, which drains mucus and in turn relieves sinus headache.

Also press:

- Stomach 36 to strengthen digestion
- Large Intestine 4 to eliminate the mucus
- Large Intestine 20, a local point to open the nose and sinuses

When we have a headache of any kind, we often find ourselves pressing our fingers to our heads. Indeed, acupressure—and using specific points—is a great way to relieve headaches. In my practice, the most common acupoint I use to treat headaches is Large Intestine 4. Headaches concentrate in different parts of the head. The following is a list of the areas where you might experience headache pain, the imbalanced organs causing it, and the points to treat:

- under the occipital bone at the back of the head (bladder), Gallbladder 20
- forehead and cheek region (stomach), Gallbladder 14 and Stomach 3
- temples (Gallbladder), *taiyang* and Gallbladder 34
- sides of the head, especially on the left (liver), Large Intestine 4 and Liver 3

Note: When you have a terrible headache, it's hard not to frown. The nice thing about the combination of points above is that they are also very effective points for a natural face-lift—sure to put a smile back on your face!

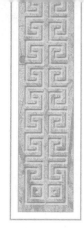

Hearing Problems

WHEN my patients have problems with hearing, whether deafness, partial hearing loss, clogged ears, or ringing in their ears (tinnitus), I look to the kidneys and the liver. The kidneys nourish the ears, and deficiency in the kidneys is responsible for hearing loss. The liver may become irritated by a flaring of fire disturbing the ears that leads to tinnitus. Treatment is focused on either strengthening the liver and kidneys to counteract a deficient condition such as hearing loss or calming liver energy to counteract an excessive condition such as a banging, clanging, persistent ringing, or buzzing in the ears.

Qigong movements to improve hearing include:

- Beating the Heavenly Drum
- Spinning Wheel
- Rag Doll Twist
- Swan Stretches Her Wings

Self-acupressure on local points to improve hearing:

- Small Intestine 19
- Triple Warmer 21
- Gallbladder 2
- Large Intestine 20 and Stomach 3 if caused by sinus problems

Other self-acupressure points for ear health:

- Small intestine 3
- Stomach 44 specifically for ear ringing

Strengthen kidneys with:

- The Kidney Rub for Life (page 103)
- Healing Sound for Kidneys thirty-six times

Remember that the kidneys hate cold, so please avoid raw, cold foods, ice in drinks, walking barefoot on cold floors, and allowing cold wind to hit your lower back. When it comes to food, the kidneys are nourished by naturally salty foods such as tomatoes, chicken, fish, and lamb, and by black or dark blue foods such as black beans, black sesame seeds, plums, and walnuts.

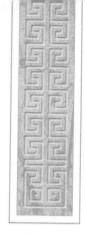

High/Low Blood Pressure

HIGH BLOOD PRESSURE

Qigong has been proven to control and even eliminate high blood pressure, and you may well see results of this kind after you begin your practice. Very high blood pressue is dangerous. Please don't go it alone! If you have high blood pressure, it is essential that you ask your physician to work with you when you are ready to bring it down with natural means. If you are on medication and begin practicing qigong, make sure to check your blood pressure on a regular basis, because your pressure may come down. Your doctor can help you to reduce your medication at the appropriate time and/or monitor you in a safe way.

The organs associated with high blood pressure include the heart, kidneys, liver, and stomach. Depending on your individual pattern, it could be that there is an excess fire condition of the heart ultimately resulting from kidney deficiency. Or an inadequacy of the stomach could also be the culprit, interfering with the heart's ability to properly pump blood through the entire system. Additionally, it could be that you have excessive fire of the liver (stemming from deficiency of kidneys), which has stirred the fire of the heart.

Due to the interaction of all of these organ systems, to treat high blood pressure, practice the Twenty-Minute Workout in its entirety. This applies to high cholesterol levels as well.

When our bodies are under pressure, we may become easily overexcited. Some people with excessive heart fire laugh during almost every interaction with others. A little laughter relieves pressure in your system, but excessive laughing builds pressure on the heart. Be careful about perspiration during exercise since an excessive amount can weaken the qi of the heart. Practice the following specific exercises in the workout to lower blood pressure:

- Back Swinging Monkey
- Swan Stretches Her Wings
- Energize Endocrines for Adrenal Glands
- Spinning Wheel

Use the following acupressure points to relieve high blood pressure:

- Gall bladder 20 and Liver 3 to balance the liver
- Kidney 3 to strengthen kidney qi
- Large Intestine 11 and Stomach 36 to nourish digestion

In Chinese dietary therapy there are a host of foods eaten to help high blood pressure. Some of these include garlic, tofu, watermelon, sunflower seeds, bananas, and celery. Three cups of celery juice per day is the recommended dosage for treating hypertension.

LOW BLOOD PRESSURE

Low blood pressure stems from a deficiency of blood or from having not enough qi to move blood. Improperly directed qi can prevent blood *and* qi from nourishing the head and the extremities. This, in turn, has an ill effect on immune function and ability for proper nourishment. Practice the entire Twenty-Minute Workout to build blood and raise qi to remedy this situation.

The following acupoints will also help:

- Stomach 36 and Spleen 6 to build blood
- Pericardium 6 regulates the flow of qi
- Governing Vessel 25, treats low blood pressure
- Large Intestine 4 and Large Intestine 11 to bolster the immune system

The declining strength of kidney energy that comes with aging makes a woman more susceptible to problems with her heart because, according to the five-element theory, the kidneys control the heart. This provides even more compelling impetus for the ageless women to practice qigong to preserve, consolidate, nurture, and cultivate her kidney qi.

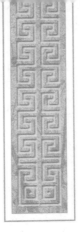

Hot Flashes

BEFORE the age of forty, depending on her individual constitution, a woman normally exhibits either deficiency of the yin (water) of the kidneys or deficiency of the yang (fire) of the kidneys. During menopausal years, women usually have *both* yin and yang deficiency of the kidneys combined with blood deficiency. These deficiencies are at the root of many women's health problems during and after menopause, including hot flashes. Hot flashes that stem from kidney deficiency are usually accompanied by dryness of the eyes and skin.

We have dryness accompanied by hot flashes when the deficiency of yin in the kidneys is so severe that it creates something called empty or false heat. One of the maxims of the yin-yang theory is that an excess of yin turns into yang and vice versa. Whenever we have a severe deficiency, our body overcompensates by switching to its opposite condition: excess. When there is so great a deficiency of fluids, our body creates an excess of fire. This empty heat is usually a result of extreme loss of blood or of water, resulting in an inability to dampen and control fire within the woman's system.

After the age of sixty, a woman's predominant deficiency (either yin or yang) becomes more and more pronounced. If she was yin deficient before menopause, she becomes more so after menopause, and yin begins to over-shadow yang in her system. If she has been yang deficient, yang will continue to decrease in her system. This explains why some women stop having hot flashes and others continue to have them for many years after their menstrual cycle stops.

Whether you have hot flashes for one week or ten years, during the day or at night, they can be a great annoyance during the menopausal years. There is no known cure for hot flashes, but it may help you through them to think of them as creative power surges. Accept them as best you can, for they are a part of our transition as our hormones get rearranged, a right of passage of sorts. You can control their frequency and intensity. The best qigong exercises to soothe hot flashes are:

- Walking Like a Turtle
- Woman Connects with Heaven and Earth
- Lady Raises Lotus to the Temple
- Fluffing White Clouds
- Practicing sending appreciation to all of your endocrine glands as part of the Energize Endocrines set.

Use the following acupressure points to cool down and thus alleviate night sweats:

- Triple Warmer 5
- Large Intestine 4 combined with Large Intestine 11
- Kidney 3
- Small Intestine 3

It is especially important for the ageless woman to keep her lower back and *mingmen* point (see illustration page 81) at the area of her kidneys warm. Warmth allows optimal functioning of the kidneys and adrenals. The thought of creating more warmth in between hot flashes and especially after hot flashes have stopped is the last thing many of us want to do. Even so, it's important to do so to the best of your ability, as not keeping the fire of the kidneys stoked can bring a host of other problems.

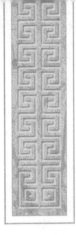

Insomnia

IT IS COMPLETELY normal to experience insomnia during the menopausal years. The organ keeping us up at night is the liver. The liver stores most of the blood in the body. When the blood of the liver is deficient, as it often can be when women grow older, it leads to insomnia because there is not enough blood to nourish the head. Our thoughts go round and round, keeping us awake long after we are tired. In addition, when there is deficient blood of the liver, there is also deficiency of yin, or water, in the kidneys, often to such an extent that it leads to a flaring of fire. A deficiency of the heart and spleen can further complicate the matter by not producing enough blood, leading to palpitations. And a lack of harmony between the kidneys and heart adds the component of mental restlessness.

The following qigong exercises promote restful sleep:

- Healing Sounds for Liver, Kidneys, Heart, and Spleen
- Rag Doll Twist

- Separating Clouds
- Swan Stretches Her Wings

For a good night's rest, you may also practice:

- Energize Endocrines for Hypothalamus and Pineal Glands
- Back Swinging Monkey
- Fluffing White Clouds

For self-acupressure:

- Urinary Bladder 62 is the acupoint of choice for insomnia. It can be pressed during the day for prevention or you can do this point on both ankles in the middle of the night.
- Spleen 6, where the liver, spleen, and kidney meridians cross, balances all three of these meridians to help reduce or eliminate insomnia.

The following suggestions for insomnia can be done alone or in combination. Obviously, if the first one works you will stay asleep! You may find that one works one night and another one works the next night. Experiment. If you've gone through all of them and you are still awake, start the cycle over again.

RESTFUL SLUMBER REPERTOIRE

From the point of view of Chinese medicine, the Hundred Meeting point, located at the crown of your head, is the area to focus on for treating insomnia. Hundred Meeting point is located along with a combination of four points called *sishencong*. Both are where all the yang meridians converge in the body. Hundred Meeting point is treated to clear the senses, calm the spirit, and stabilize mental disorders. *Sishencong* is treated to resolve nervousness, headache, vertigo, and insomnia.

To treat insomnia, soothe this area by lying down and placing one hand on the top of your head. Sometimes, this alone can calm your mind down enough for you to sleep. For many of you who experience insomnia, hundreds

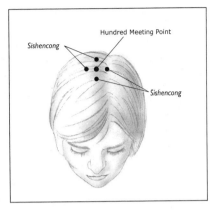

Sishencong

Hundred Meeting Point

Sishencong

● *Hundred Meeting Point*

of thoughts are flooding into your mind from above. So as you lie with your hand on your head, visualize warm, fuzzy feelings surrounding your crown, providing you with the love, comfort, and calm that is holding you in just the exact way you need to go off into a sweet slumber. Do this from five to fifteen minutes or more until you doze off.

You can also treat your insomnia with a *sishencong* qi massage. Use a circular motion, spiraling outward about two inches from the top center of your head. When doing this exercise you can also put your other hand on your belly, on your *dantian* (3 to 5 minutes). This helps you to ground yourself more into your body, which settles you down and also helps induce sleep.

You will be able to stop thoughts swirling endlessly and go to sleep by visualizing your thousand thoughts transforming into one. If this doesn't work and you still feel bombarded by thoughts and concerns about others, place your hand over your *dantian* to ground and control the heart energy by stimulating and strengthening the kidneys. Next, put your other hand gently over your nose and allow your fingertips to cover the place between your eyebrows. Do for five to ten minutes to help you drift off. This acupoint between your eyebrows is called *yintang* (see illustration page 159). It calms your heart and spirit and releases feelings of being suspended in midair as you lie there thinking.

Massage the *mingmen* point (see illustration on page 81) on your lower back, which strengthens the kidneys to induce sleep. This point is located between your kidneys and above your sacrum and directly behind your belly button. Make a loose fist and massage yourself there with a circular motion thirty times one direction and thirty times the opposite direction (30 seconds). This circular qi massage on your lower back treats insomnia by bringing your spirit home and refocusing scattered qi. Do count the circles as you make them, as this often brings sleep before you know it—I call this counting qi! While counting, be strict with your mind and don't allow it to wander. When you finish, rest your hand by your side. You will most likely feel calmer and sense the energy sinking lower to your center of gravity. If you are still awake after a few minutes, repeat the exercise. Afterward, rest your hand by your side and notice the sensations. If you don't feel yourself drifting off after a few minutes, repeat the massage. Sometimes I wake up my husband and ask him to do the circles for me. I don't feel bad and he doesn't mind since *he* has no problem going back to sleep!

If the third time doesn't do it, start over again with the first exercise, touching the Hundred Meeting point and your *dantian* simultaneously. Follow steps one to three repeatedly until you drift off into restful sleep.

OTHER TIPS ‖

- Try mugwort pillows, easily found in health food stores and also called dream pillows, to help ward off bad dreams that wake us from sleep.
- Don't eat too much late at night.
- If you just can't go to sleep or get back to sleep, don't fight it. Consider getting out of bed to write in a journal or read a book—maybe your subconscious mind is telling you something. Sometimes the quality of your sleep is more important than the quantity.

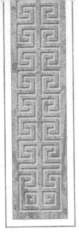

Leg Cramps/Spasms

PRACTICING the entire Twenty-Minute Workout will naturally help relieve leg cramps. Leg cramps stem from problems with the circulatory system, which is intricately connected with the respiratory system. When your breathing is hindered, so is the free flow of blood through your body. The continuous, gentle movements of qigong increase the flow of oxygen by moving clean blood throughout the body, thus preventing cramps and spasms in the legs.

Concentrate on Woman Connects with Heaven and Earth to strengthen the blood circulation in your legs.

The girdle vessel stands on its own as the only horizontal meridian in the body. It encircles the main meridians and exerts an influence on the circulation of qi to the legs. Practice of the following exercises promotes flow of qi within the girdle vessel:

- Beautiful Woman Turns at Hips
- Feeling Qi
- Standing Like a Tree Posture 8

For extra help with leg cramps, do self-acupressure. If you can catch the leg cramp or spasm before it happens, quickly press Governing Vessel 26 (see illustration page 159), located on the center of the indentation between your nose and your lip. Take your finger and press this point with as much pressure as you can stand. Press deeply into the spot over the place where the top of your front teeth meets your gums. Using the tip of your thumb works well. After pressing this point, quickly grab the part of your leg that is in spasm and massage it deeply. Do acupressure on the center of the spasming muscle and continue until the tight, tender spot goes away. If you act quickly in the moment you sense it coming on you should be able to avoid a muscle cramp or spasm altogether. Also try Large Intestine 4 for leg cramps.

Remember to also eat one banana per day. The potassium in bananas helps prevent the onset of muscle cramps. Eating enough foods containing calcium also helps. You can get calcium naturally from green leafy vegetables, sesame seeds, canned sardines or salmon with bones, yogurt, and tofu.

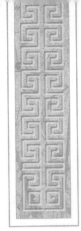

Menstration, Conception, and Other Gynecological Issues

WOMEN are all about blood. When it comes to menstruation and other gynecological issues, all of our organs, especially the spleen, liver, heart, and kidneys, are involved in the quality and quantity of blood in our systems. Your particular issues may stem more from one than another. No matter the root, the organs are intricately connected, especially as they influence the penetrating and girdle vessels that support the female reproductive system.

The quality and quantity of a woman's kidney essence has a tremendous impact on her gynecological health during all phases of her life. *Jing*, the source of life, provides for reproduction, growth, and development throughout a woman's life cycle. It is found in ovarian eggs, bone marrow, and the brain and is stored in our kidneys. The kidneys are a source of both water and fire and influence the uterus, which stores the blood. During the menopausal years, both the water and fire aspects of the kidneys become deficient. To promote menstrual regularity and gynecological health, we must care for our kidneys and our kidney *jing*.

There are many exercises in the Twenty-Minute Workout that focus attention and move energy in the *dantian*, thus strengthening the kidneys and uterus. The following are recommended for gynecological health:

- Standing Like a Tree posture 3 and 4
- Fluffing White Clouds
- Rag Doll Twist
- Walking Like a Turtle

The Kidney Rub for Life (page 103) helps to build the fire of the kidneys, affects menstruation, and warms the uterus, promoting conception.

The girdle vessel is used to treat abnormal menstruation and is a way to stimulate both the essence and the fire of the kidneys. The following exercises are practiced to open the flow of energy in the girdle vessel. When you do these exercises, use your mind to send the intent of healing energy there.

- Beautiful Woman Turns at Hips
- Feeling Qi
- Standing Like a Tree posture 8

The heart governs blood and houses the mind, so when not enough heart blood is present, a woman tends to become overly pensive and worried. Sadness leads to the stagnation of blood, which manifests in painful periods, irregular menstruation, lack of menstruation, or vaginal pain and itching. This can occur when we are overworking, experiencing mental strain and too much stress. Lady Raises Lotus to the Temple stimulates flow of heart energy and blood.

Due to its relationship with the uterus and blood, the liver is also of great importance in gynecological health. When the blood (yin aspect) of the liver is deficient, it leads to problems with menstruation such as irregular and scanty periods, delayed cycle, or lack of period. Additionally, when the qi (yang, fire aspect) of the liver is stagnant or rising, this can create menstrual clotting, headaches before or during menses, painful periods, premenstrual tension, irritability, depression, and abdominal bloating and pain. Because the uterus is located in the lower abdomen and stores blood, women are extremely vulnerable to stagnation of blood in the abdominal area. Because the liver moves qi and blood, one of the most commonly occurring patterns is liver qi stagnation.

The following exercises promote health of the liver meridian:

- Healing Sound for Liver
- Rag Doll Twist
- Separating Clouds
- Swan Stretches Her Wings

Menstrual blood is derived from the qi extracted from food. The digestive role of the spleen plays an important role in painful menstruation. It results from deficiency of qi and blood, due to insufficient amounts of each derived from the essence of food. The spleen keeps blood flowing in the vessels, preventing conditions such as uterine prolapse, rectal prolapse, dropped stomach, or dropped intestines. Additionally, when the spleen is deficient, it may not build enough blood and this can lead to deficient blood of the liver.

Much depends, too, on the stomach and on eating properly, keys to healthy menstruation. Problems with the stomach energy can also lead to morning sickness, nausea, and premenstrual tension. Deficiency of the lungs may lead to worry, grief, and sadness that can indirectly create a loss of period or premenstrual tension, breast distention, breathlessness, and sighing. Swan Stretches Her Wings is an excellent qigong exercise to address root causes.

When women have problems associated with menstruation, infertility, and spasms in the abdominal region, attention must be paid to the three meridians that connect with the uterus. They are the penetrating vessel, which controls qi and is used to strengthen and nourish blood, the conception vessel, which controls blood and is used to move qi and blood and remove obstructions, and the governing vessel, which controls the life gate fire and the minister fire and is used to maintain a good balance between qi and blood.

As the Sea of Blood, the penetrating vessel moves blood to the uterus, which controls menstruation and breaks up blood and qi stagnation, which promotes health of the entire body. As mentioned previously in the section on breast health, an energetic connection exists between the penetrating vessel and the uterus. To strengthen the penetrating vessel and create free flow of qi and blood to resolve stagnation, do acupressure on:

- Spleen 4
- Pericardium 6

Practice Monkey Stretches Up and Down and Phoenix Eats Its Ashes to promote a healthy gynecological system. Both strengthen the governing vessel that provides minister fire, the special fire that moistens rather than dries the body.

Practicing the Microcosmic Orbit (page 198) is another way to open the flow of qi within the governing vessel. This exercise also opens the flow within the conception vessel. This vessel is associated with abnormal menstruation and pain in the lower abdomen. You can also do acupressure on Conception Vessel 6 and Spleen 6 to strengthen the conception vessel, help promote normal menstruation, and eliminate pain in the lower abdomen.

FERTILITY

I have a lot to say about this subject since I treat many women for fertility, particularly women over thirty-five. Often, they have been told by doctors that their eggs are old and their systems are withering. First, I ask them not to succumb to any negative belief about their bodies. By seeing yourself as vibrant, juicy, healthy, with a warm, open, and fertile womb, visualizing all of this during your qigong practice, you can personally disprove society's views (or your doctor's, your mother's, and so on).

Difficulties conceiving often have to do with coldness, a condition that can be reversed. When too cold, a woman does not possess enough blood to nourish her own body, let alone a fetus. When blood of the liver is deficient, the uterus can become invaded by cold because it doesn't have enough blood. When the uterus is obstructed by cold, the blood of the liver can't be properly stored, leading to more blood deficiency and thus more coldness. This can be a vicious cycle. To become pregnant after the age of thirty-five, it is important to strengthen liver blood and release liver qi stagnation.

Deficiency of the yang of the kidneys, common as we age, is important to reverse. Deficiency of kidney yin that relates to *jing,* or essence, is another crucial factor. Without an abundant amount of *jing,* which is the "juice" of reproduction, conception may be challenged.

It is of utmost importance to reduce stress, get ample sleep, balance work and play, have regular, healthy eating habits, and protect your kidney energy at all costs. Since we get *jing* from the food and water we take in, I always advise women not to diet while attempting to conceive. Additionally, I recommend that they temper their intake of cold and iced food to avoid coldness of the uterus. Limit consumption of greasy foods and dairy because these can lead to dampness in their lower abdomen. Both excessive coldness and dampness may prevent fertilization. Based upon my experience helping women to become mothers, I have found it to be essential to build the systems with a nutritious array of well-balanced, high-quality food and drinks.

Additionally, liver stagnation or constraint creates tension within a woman's energetic system, which can block sperm from reaching the ovum. This goes hand in hand with the old adage passed on by our grandmothers that in order to conceive, we need to relax. I always tell my fertility patients to go on a vacation during their fertile times. All three of my own children were conceived on vacation—two Borscht Belt babies and one in Mexico! I encourage women to hope that they can and will conceive, recommending that they be around as many babies as possible and visit stores to look at baby clothes.

Mature women can and do become pregnant. I was thirty-nine for my first, and forty-four for my third! I believe the jury is still out regarding the risk of having children when older; there just has not been enough of us doing it until now. It is essential that a woman, no matter what age, find the right pregnancy and labor support team to champion her fertility. With this faith, support, and hope, along with the power qigong instills, you will realize your dreams.

Acupoint suggestions:

- Liver 3 releases stagnation of liver energy
- Gallbladder 34 benefits the liver
- Stomach 36 combined with Spleen 6 to build blood
- Pericardium 6 combined with Spleen 4 to open the penetrating vessel
- Gallbladder 41 combined with Triple Warmer 5 to open the girdle vessel

Qigong for promoting fertility:

- Kidney Rub for Life on page 103 to spark kidney yang
- Lady Carries Lotus to the Temple to harmonize *jing*, qi, and *shen*
- Fluffing White Clouds to open qi flow throughout the body
- Walking Like a Turtle to strengthen mind and body
- Standing Like a Tree to nourish kidneys and balance yin and yang
- Ovarian Triangle exercise on page 232 to nourish the uterus, clitoris, and ovaries
- Energize Endocrine exercises to promote hormone secretion
- Horse Stance (page 11) to strengthen the girdle vessel

Helpful Hint

After intercourse, lie on your back and bring your hips up into the air to bring the semen down into your womb. You may want to place a pillow under yourself for comfort. Instead of staying in that position all by your-self (how unromantic!) ask your partner to sit behind you so you are back-to-back. Lie this way and visualize the sperm going where it needs to go. As you connect back-to-back take deep, slow, gentle, and rhythmic breaths together and visualize a precious little being coming into your womb to share your lives with you (3 to 5 minutes).

FIBROID TUMORS AND OVARIAN CYSTS

Abdominal masses such as uterine fibroids and ovarian cysts come from stagnation of qi and blood of the liver. This stagnation also causes painful menstrual periods with dark blood and clots and premenstrual pain (which goes away once menstrual bleeding begins). Estrogen feeds fibroids, so thanks to declining estrogen levels, uterine fibroids usually shrink on their own once women reach menopause. If you have fibroids or a tendency toward them, practice Swan Stretches Her Wings to balance the energy within the liver meridian and the Horse Stance (page 11) to stimulate the flow of qi and blood in the abdominal area and girdle vessel.

Use acupressure on Kidney 6 located on the ankle, which treats the reproductive system or the lower abdomen, especially masses and fibroids.

For general gynecological health or for a specific issue like fibroids, practice the Ovarian Triangle Exercise (1 to 2 minutes) for the uterus and ovaries. The breathing technique for this exercise is called the Reverse Breathing Method, which is the opposite of natural breathing. This means that when you inhale contract your belly and when you exhale expand your belly. This type of breathing stimulates the flow of qi in your uterus and ovaries and strengthens the yang (fire) energy of the body. The uterus is intimately related to the *dantian,* and reversed breathing stimulates the health of this area.

Begin the exercise by forming a triangle with your hands. Touching the tips of your thumbs and the tips of each of your fingertips together, place this triangle close to, but not touching, your lower abdomen, index fingers pointed down. Focus your mind to send healing energy to your uterus and ovaries. Visualize vibrant, clean qi moving into your uterus and ovaries upon inhalation. Imagine any toxins or negative energy leaving your uterus and ovaries upon exhalation. If you have a growth in this area, see it dissolving and leaving your body upon exhalation.

Energize Endocrine for the Ovaries Exercise (repeated thirty-six times) also gives extra special attention to the ovaries. As the hormones are at the basis of every gynecological stage and transition for a woman, doing all of the exercises in this set enhances the gynecological system.

UTERINE PROLAPSE

For prolapse of the uterus, which comes from qi deficiency of the lungs and the spleen, strengthen the girdle vessel to keep it relaxed and stretched, but not too slack. When slack, the organs sag, causing prolapse and, in pregnancy, miscarriage. The following exercises stimulate qi in the girdle vessel:

- Beautiful Woman Turns at Hips
- Feeling Qi
- Standing Like a Tree Posture 8

Press Hundred Meeting point to eliminate the possibility of recurrence of uterine prolapse.

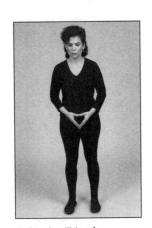

● *Ovarian Triangle*

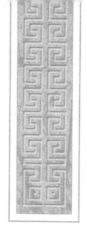

Mental Clarity/Good Memory

THE ANCIENT Chinese medical text *Yellow Emperor's Classic* states that when the brain is functioning properly and in good condition, the aging process is slowed. A healthy brain can be achieved through qigong exercises that send qi to the brain. This is essential to a calm and peaceful mind because one must regulate emotions to stay centered mentally. The heart houses the mind. In order for the mind to be properly nourished, the heart blood must be plentiful. Deficiency of both the heart blood and the spleen qi lead to poor memory. Depletion of liver blood and stagnation of liver qi also cause memory problems and obstruct the mind.

Proper nutrition is an important element for mental clarity. Follow the basic suggestions below to nourish your body, and thereby, your mind:

- Sour or green foods nourish the liver.
- Sweet yellow or orange foods nourish the spleen.
- Bitter or red foods nourish the heart, such as horseradish, watermelon, beets, red apples.

Beating the Heavenly Drum Variation

Beating the Heavenly Drum is the best exercise for promoting brain power and optimal mental health. After you are finished with Beating the Heavenly Drum, gently massage your scalp using a circular kneading motion followed by gentle tapping. This will stimulate the acupressure points located on the scalp and perk up your mental faculties. After completing this qi massage, take a moment to concentrate your mind's eye on the crown of your head. Visualize bright healing energy coming into this point from the heavens above. Then take your hand and, touching the top of your head, make three clockwise circles and then three counterclockwise circles. End this exercise by gently placing your hands on your belly and taking three deep, rhythmic breaths into your *dantian*. Keep your eyes open for the duration of this exercise. It can be done in a seated or standing position. This stimulates the four points called *sishencong* as well as Hundred Meeting point located on the top of your head. This takes about one minute if combined with Beating the Heavenly Drum.

The brain, bone, and marrow are closely associated in Chinese medicine and are always associated with and treated through the kidneys. The Bone Marrow Washing exercises can also be done to nourish the brain.

Treating the heart is also essential for keeping the mind's "house" peaceful and orderly. The kidneys control the heart and the heart controls the mind. When the kidneys are weakened, fear ensues, clouding the clarity of the mind. The heart is also equated with the *shen* or spiritual aspect of our being. A balanced heart provides enough blood and qi to create a healthy mind and spirit. If there isn't adequate heart blood the spirit is restless rather than peaceful, the body is agitated rather than relaxed, and your mental power is waning rather than waxing. Practice Healing Sound for Heart to bolster mental clarity. Always remember that the heart and mind are one. Chinese medicine views the mind as more powerful than the body in relationship to a person's emotional, spiritual, and physical health.

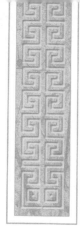

Sexual Dysfunction

SEX IS a funny animal, isn't it? Some women have strong sexual desire throughout their lives no matter what, while others have a waxing and waning drive depending on hormone activity. Still others have been "nearly dead" sexually for as long as they can remember. For many women, sexual activity changes depending upon their stage of life and it's no surprise that many women couldn't care less about sex during the menopausal years.

If you so desire, however, the menopausal years can prove to be the best years of your life when it comes to sex. Don't get carried away—too much sex drains qi from the kidneys and we need all the kidney qi we can get for a healthy back, strong knees, clear mind, and long, vital life. When it comes to sex in the second half of your life, think quality, not quantity.

Lack of desire for sex can come from a lack of fire or yang of the kidneys, which can be accompanied by a feeling of coldness or lassitude. Stoke the fire of your kidneys with the Kidney Rub for Life (page 103). This can be practiced once or twice a day and helps to promote the energy of your kidneys, giving you more fire for love.

The heart energy also has to do with lovemaking because it provides within us a fire or passion for others and the desire to connect with another human being in an intimate way. We need to cultivate and care for our heart fire, saving it for those special times of physical sharing with our significant other. Practice Lady Raises Lotus to the Temple and Healing Sound for Heart to nourish your heart. Laugh and find humor in life.

Sexual energy also comes from good blood flow from the liver. Keep your frustrations and anger flowing out of your mouth in an appropriate manner rather than keeping a lid on them. Releasing these emotions, in turn, releases blockages that can accumulate in the liver meridian. Shaking the Tree (page 165) releases these blockages. This spontaneous qigong form allows you to intuitively and creatively shake your body in whatever way moves you. In so doing, you release blockages in your joints, in your spine, and in your connective tissue. It also helps to bring that sweet inner smile on your face as you shake your way to freedom and health.

The menopausal years are a great time to really enjoy yourself sexually. One benefit of empty nests is that we don't have to worry about the children barging in. After menopause, we don't have to worry about getting pregnant, and ideally we are experiencing greater love for ourselves than ever before. All of these things allow us to enjoy more fully the simple pleasures of sex.

Whether you think of sex as good exercise, a way to commune with your higher spiritual nature, a way to share love with your special someone, or just a nice way to spend your time, I encourage you to enjoy it. It's healthy for your body, keeping your sexual organs healthy by creating movement there. And if you don't have someone special to share sex with, engage in masturbation. Give your clitoris the attention it needs. These parts of your body need exercise just like any other. As we tend to get drier with passing years, massage oils and organic creams can help with lubrication (see the section on dryness if this is an issue).

There are three major vessels that go through the girdle vessel, which are interlinked and have a profound affect on production, circulation, discharge, and regeneration of sexual energy. They are the governing vessel going up the back center, the conception vessel going up the front center, and the penetrating vessel going up the middle of your torso. These meridians link the heart with the genital system. When these meridians are blocked, sexual energy also becomes blocked.

For more sexual energy, practice the following exercises to promote energy flow in the girdle vessel:

- Beautiful Woman Turns at Hips
- Fluffing White Clouds
- Feeling Qi
- Standing Like a Tree posture 8
- Energize Endocrines for Ovaries can also be done to enhance sexual energy. You can smile into and thus stimulate this area to bring more qi and blood to your ovaries, vagina, clitoris, and uterus. As you smile into this area make sure to give the area your love and appreciation for giving you the gift of life, making hormones, providing excitement along with pleasure, and providing you with ample sexual energy.

Acupressure points for improving sexual health:

- Conception Vessel 6
- Liver 9
- Kidney 3

❀ Ovarian Qigong Exercise *(7 minutes, 30 seconds)*

Ovarian breathing practices can be helpful during menopause. The following breathing exercises will help you recycle sexual energy into a qi "reservoir" that you can dip into on a daily basis to create whatever it is you want and need in your life. These breathing techniques are part of a wider set of practices called Taoist sexual practices. They are ultimately employed at advanced levels of practice to transform your *jing* (sexual essence) into *shen* to reach higher levels of awareness. These practices promote a greater connection between your heart energy and your sexual energy. They also instill more control over your sexual desires.

Ovarian breathing practices ignite and rekindle sexual energy. They recycle sexual energy into your *dantian.* Remember, your uterus is intimately related to your *dantian*. Vibrant and plentiful energy within your uterus helps you to get through the challenges and stress of daily life. It provides you with excitement not only on a sexual basis but also for creating what it is you want and need in your life.

Sit comfortably on a chair with your back straight, head erect, and chin relaxed. Your brow is soft and relaxed, your mouth closed, and your tongue rests on the roof of your mouth. With your feet flat on the floor and hands on your lap, begin by drawing your attention to your perineum point (page 174). As you slowly inhale, gently contract the muscles of your perineum, tighten your sphincter muscles, and tilt your pelvis forward as you imagine yourself grasping sexual energy from your ovaries. Next, visualize yourself bringing this sexual energy from your ovaries up along the center of your back all the way up to Hundred Meeting point on the crown of your head.

Begin your exhalation as you visualize a spiraling pattern around the crown of your head. Continue this visualization for several breaths and then sit quietly for a moment to take in the feelings. When ready, first inhale and then exhale as you follow your attention down the front centerline of your body to your *dantian* (about 1 minute).

You can repeat this cycle up to a total of six times. Just make sure that on your last cycle, you leave out the visualization of grasping sexual energy from your ovaries to prevent stuck qi from being left in your energetic system. Without this part of the visualization you are essentially doing the Microcosmic Orbit exercise (approximately 6 minutes).

At the conclusion of this exercise, place your right hand on your belly. Cover your right hand with your left hand and circle your hands around your belly three times clockwise and three times counterclockwise. Make small circles. This consolidates and stores your qi in your *dantian*.

URINATION PROBLEMS/BLADDER PROLAPSE

If you are running to the bathroom to urinate constantly, not able to urinate when you get the urge, or not able to get to the bathroom in time, there are several solutions. Incontinence can occur when we are undergoing a lot of stress or when we have an infection, but most bladder problems we experience when older stem from a deficiency of kidney yin (water) and yang (fire).

In Chinese medicine, another source of incontinence is coldness in the lower abdominal region. Treatments that warm the pelvic area and strengthen the muscles that hold up pelvic floor muscles are very effective. During qigong, concentrate on your *dantian* to produce the warmth your body needs to expel excess water and purify your urine.

The best way to treat incontinence is through the stimulation of the conception vessel through practice of the Microcosmic Orbit (page 198).

For both retention of urine and incontinence, do self-acupressure on:

- Spleen 9
- Liver 9
- Kidney 3

If you find yourself urinating too frequently, practice the following visualization exercise (about 1 minute):

Lie on your back with your knees bent and your feet flat on the floor near your buttocks. Place your hands on your *dantian*. Breathe deeply through your nose, keeping your mouth closed and your tongue relaxed at the top of your mouth. Visualize a dark blue color emanating from your hands, moving into your lower abdomen and surrounding your bladder. Massage yourself with this color, strengthening the area so that it functions at its very best.

Like prolapse of the uterus, prolapse of the bladder occurs when the organ drops down and even needs to be surgically lifted. This is known as collapsed qi and results from qi deficiency of the lungs and the spleen. The lungs govern qi and the spleen is responsible for holding things up and in their place. The girdle vessel raises spleen qi and nourishes descending qi. The girdle vessel needs to remain relaxed and stretched, but when the girdle vessel is too slack, the bladder sags, causing prolapse. The following exercises stimulate qi in the girdle vessel and can be done to prevent or treat prolapse of the bladder. When you practice these, visualize them making your bladder healthier and stronger:

- Beautiful Woman Turns at Hips
- Feeling Qi
- Standing Like a Tree posture 8

Pressing Hundred Meeting point is a wonderful and effective way to help the vital organs in your body stay in place, counteracting the drooping created as gravity pulls down on them. Your body must counteract that pull with vibrant, vital, and abundant yang qi stimulated at this point.

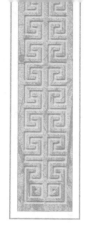

Weight and Food Issues

THE MENOPAUSAL years are accompanied by sudden changes in metabolism and hormones. Pounds that once dropped off in a few days no longer shed so easily but instead stick like glue. As women, we can sometimes obsess about food and weight, getting distracted from doing what we really need to do in our later years. This is a time of great potential for us if we can only decide how to make use of it and realize our calling. When we discover what it is that's "eating at us" we can often change what we are eating.

Each woman has her own unique food issues: overconsumption of the right foods; underconsumption of healthy food combined with junk-food eating; emotional bingeing on refined sugar; overindulging in fatty, fried, salty snacks; or some other unhealthy pattern of eating. As with so many health challenges, qi is key.

Qigong can help with your food and weight issues in many ways, including strengthening your willpower, eliminating cravings, quickening metabolism, and providing better access to the qi of the foods you eat.

When qi is flowing effervescently, your body reinforces this qi flow, allowing you to maintain a healthy weight. The organ that governs digestion in Oriental medicine is the spleen, which is responsible for the transformation and transportation of food. Problems with weight come first and foremost from problems with digestive energy derived from the spleen. If food is not properly transformed and transported to the tissues, cells, and organs, then food, fluid, and mucus become stagnant, leading to excess weight. This creates a damp condition of the spleen, and the spleen definitely doesn't like dampness. When the energy of the spleen is balanced through qigong, your body digests food better and a shift in your weight will occur. Spleen qi depletion comes from a poorly functioning digestive system that can't transform and transport the food. Our spleen qi can be depleted due to excess anger, stress, drinking too much water, eating too much or too little and too late in the day, and eating rich or processed foods.

Qi flow is very important in relationship to metabolism. Practicing your Twenty-Minute Workout on an empty stomach can quicken your metabolic rate. Hormonal levels are also a key factor with how you store and process your food. Stimulate your hormonal system by practicing the Energize Endocrine exercise.

If you overeat because you feel disconnected emotionally and spiritually, it could be caused by a disturbance of your *shen*. When you practice qigong and choose healthier foods, your *shen* is clearer and brighter. As you do your qigong and combine it with an open and positive attitude, you enhance your spiritual awareness, improve your cerebral function, and follow a path of higher spiritual work. Practice Lady Raises Lotus to the Temple and Lifting Qi Ball to help build your *shen*.

The Chinese believe that our body is formed out of an essence derived from the foods we eat. The special qi that comes from the food we eat is called gu qi, which sounds a lot like the noise we make for babies. Maybe it's no coincidence! Getting good gu qi is how we baby ourselves. The qi in what we eat is essential for our overall health, beauty, and well-being. Qi provides the basic nourishment and energy that activates the entire system. Its potency depends on the quality of food and water consumed and the efficiency of our digestive system. If we eat poor-quality foods and our digestive system is not strong, gu qi will not be there to nourish our body. Qi depletion occurs from a diet that is too rich (heavy sauces, organ meats, too sweet), too fatty, too spicy, non-nutritious (sugar, caffeine, processed foods, alcohol), or lacking in vital quality (overcooked, filled with coloring agents and preservatives or other additives, ridden with pesticides, grown in depleted soil). Correct breathing, clean blood, and strong heart and liver functions allow for the unimpeded flow of blood and energy required for efficient delivery of nourishing energy to all parts of the body. The combination of qigong and eating right helps to make this happen.

To resolve weight issues, do self-acupressure on:

- Gallbladder 41, combined with Stomach 44
- Conception Vessel 9
- Stomach 36
- Spleen 9
- Large Intestine 11

When weight loss or gain is connected to thyroid problems, practice Energize Endocrines for Thyroid.

If you suffer from *lack* of appetite, it could be due to the accumulation of phlegm, stagnation of qi, and deficiency of the heart and spleen energy. Regain a healthy appetite by strengthening the spleen energy, promoting smooth flow of qi in the liver meridian, and nourishing the heart energy. Swan Stretches Her Wings strengthens all three of these meridian pathways. Also practice the Healing Sounds for Spleen, Heart, and Liver.

Whether by overeating or not eating enough, if we don't give ourselves the proper amounts of food on a regular basis, serious illness can result. Food addictions are tough. Unlike alcohol or cigarettes for example, which you can give up, we all need food for life. If you do have serious problems with food, please consider consulting a health professional. If your problem is getting the best of you, the very best thing you can do for yourself is to reach out for help.

Qi cultivation through deep breathing and concentration on all three of your *dantian*s helps your mind, body, and mouth connection as it activates your metabolism, keeps your digestive system alive, enhances circulation of body fluids, charges the human spirit, and is key to shining health. All three of the *dantians* are also stimulated in the warm-down.

Lower *dantian* breathing helps to stimulate the digestive organs that promote movement of food through the body and thus encourages metabolism to be at its peak. Practice Standing Like a Tree exercise 3 and specifically breathe into your lower *dantian*.

Middle *dantian* breathing helps you become more aware of your mental and emotional state and leads to a greater feeling of being satisfied with foods, less emotional eating, and fewer reasons to eat under high stress. Practice Standing Like a Tree exercise 1 and specifically breathe into your middle *dantian*.

Upper *dantian* breathing allows you to connect with your higher goals and helps you stick to your wishes and desires around food. Practice Standing Like a Tree exercise 5 and specifically breathe into your upper *dantian*.

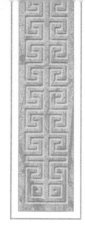

Conclusion: Becoming Ageless

So NOW you have it, a qigong book devoted to the health of women. What you do with it is up to you. Remember that a teacher can open the door for you, but it is you who needs to step across the threshold. The qi door has been opened and you have taken the first steps through. May the door lead to a beautiful, healing, empowering place for you.

I hope you feel you have learned a great deal in these pages. But know that the real knowledge comes from within yourself—your body, mind and spirit. Now you can take these movements and this knowledge and make it your own. Just watch as qi's magic manifests in your body and your life!

Practice your Twenty-Minute Workout as often as you can. If you stop for a while, don't worry. Just get back into it whenever possible. There are no shoulds here, just coulds, and the possibilities are endless. You can use this workout as your only exercise for the day or you can combine it with other forms of exercise. You can do qigong one day and your other exercises the next. Mix and match, find what works for you.

There are so many ways this book can change your life. It is dedicated to you as a balanced, peaceful, integrated woman, a woman filled with female qi power—a woman who knows and loves herself for all that she is in every way. Take this book and apply it to your life. Just as I have birthed this book, you need to birth a qigong practice within yourself. This is the essence of my teaching.

If you wish to explore the magic and wonder of qigong further, please use the resources section. There are so many qigong professionals in our midst who can help you go to the next level. All you need to do is follow your intuition and seek them out.

Qigong is not just an exercise but a way of living your life with strength, insight, flow, and gentleness. It is a way for you to be all that you want to be in life, fulfilling your greatest dreams, reaching the highest heights, creating peace and strength with all you do. Whatever it is you want, you can do it, and qigong can help you get there. It is an effective, powerful, and profound tool for a healthy, happy life. It takes commitment but you deserve to make this commitment to yourself.

I have created this guide for you and am looking forward to hearing your stories of qigong practice. Many blessings and warm regards to all of you, my qigong sisters.

Appendix: A Worksheet for Your Workout

Circle Special Additions for Your Personal Health:		
Kidney Rub for Life	Nuturing Heart	Shaking the Tree
Sunburst	Beating Sky Drum	Breathing into Beautiful Belly
Rubbing Upper Dantian	Relaxing Bowels	Great Eliminator
Fire Belly	Microcosmic Orbit	Healing Eyes
Qi Scalp Massage	Restful Slumber Repertoire	Ovarian Triangle
Beating the Heavenly Drum Variation	Ovarian Qigong	

Bibliography

Books

Ballentine, Rudolph, M.D. *Radical Healing: Integrating the World's Great Therapeutic Traditions to Create a New Transformative Medicine.* New York: Harmony Books, 1999.

Batson, Sallie and Hattie. *The Complete Idiot's Guide to Looking and Feeling Younger.* Indianapolis, IN: Alpha Books, 2000.

Baynes, Cary F., trans. *The I Ching, or Book of Changes.* Princeton, NJ: Princeton University Press, 1950.

Beinfield, Harriet, L.Ac., and Efrem Korngold, L.Ac., O.M.D. *Between Heaven and Earth: A Guide to Chinese Medicine.* New York: Ballantine Books, 1991.

Cerney, J. V. *Acupuncture without Needles: The Miracle of Chinese Healing through Your Fingertips.* New York: Cornerstone Library Publications, 1974.

Chaline, Eric. *Tai Chi: For Body, Mind and Spirit.* Ulla Weinburg, ed. New York: Sterling Publishing Company, Inc., 1998.

Chang, Stephen T. *The Book of Internal Exercises.* San Francisco: Strawberry Hill Press, 1978.

Chia, Mantak, and Maneewan Chia. *Bone Marrow Nei Kung: Taoist Ways to Improve Your Health by Rejuvenating Your Bone Marrow and Blood.* Valerie Meszaros and Charles Soupios, eds. Huntington, NY: Healing Tao Books, 1989.

Chia, Mantak, and Michael Winn. *Taoist Secrets of Love: Cultivating Male Sexual Energy.* Santa Fe, NM: Aurora Press, Inc., 1984.

Chow, David, and Richard Spanger. *Kung Fu: History, Philosophy and Technique.* Garden City, NY: Doubleday & Company, Inc., 1977.

Choy, Howard, and Belinda Henwood. *Qigong: Feng Shui for the Body.* Sydney: Macmillan Australia Pty Limited, 1998.

Clark, Angus. *The Complete Illustrated Guide to Tai Chi.* Shaftesbury, Dorset: Element Books Limited, 2000.

Cohen, Kenneth S. *The Way of Qigong: The Art and Science of Chinese Energy Healing.* New York: The Ballantine Publishing Group, 1997.

Colbin, Annemarie. *Food and Our Bones: The Natural Way to Prevent Osteoporosis.* New York: Penguin Putnam Inc., 1998.

de Lange, Jacques. *Second Book of Do-In 2: Art of Rejuvenation through Self-Massage.* Magalia, CA: Happiness Press, 1974.

De-Xin, Yan. *Aging and Blood Stasis: A New TCM Approach to Geriatrics.* Tang Guo-shun and Bob Flaws, trans. Boulder, CO: Blue Poppy Press, 1995.

Douglas, Bill. *The Complete Idiot's Guide to T'ai Chi and Qigong.* Second edition. Indianapolis, IN: Alpha Books, 2002.

East Asian Medical Studies Society. *Fundamentals of Chinese Medicine.* Brookline, MA: Paradigm Publications, 1985.

Ellis, Andrew, Nigel Wiseman, and Ken Boss. *Grasping the Wind: An Exploration into the Meaning of Chinese Acupuncture Point Names.* Brookline, MA: Paradigm Publications, 1989.

Farris, Edmond J. *Art Students' Anatomy.* New York: Dover Publications Inc., 1935.

Ferraro, Dominique. *Qigong for Women: Low-Impact Exercises for Enhancing Energy and Toning the Body.* Tami Calliope, trans. Rochester, VT: Healing Arts Press, 2000.

Flaws, Bob. *Free and Easy: Traditional Chinese Gynecology for American Women.* Boulder, CO: Blue Poppy Press, 1986.

Frantzis, B. K. *The Great Stillness,* vol. 2, The Water Method of Taoist Meditation Series. Fairfax, CA: Clarity Press, 1999.

Frantzis, B. K. *Relaxing into Your Being,* vol. 1, The Water Method of Taoist Meditation Series. Fairfax, CA: Clarity Press, 1998.

Furth, Charolette. *A Flourishing Yin: Gender in China's Medical History, 960–1665.* Berkeley, CA: University of California Press, Ltd., 1999.

Gach, Michael Reed. *Acupressure's Potent Points: A Guide to Self-Care for Common Ailments.* New York: Bantam Books, 1990.

Garripoli, Garri. *Qigong: Essence of the Healing Dance.* Deerfield Beach, FL: Health Communications, Inc., 1999.

Gaby, Alan R., M.D. *Preventing and Reversing Osteoporosis: What You Can Do about Bone Loss.* Roseville, CA: Prima Health, 1994.

Gaynor, Mitchell L. *The Healing Power of Sound: Recovery from Life-Threatening Illness Using Sound, Voice and Music.* Boston: Shambhala Publications, Inc., 1999.

Hadady, Letha, D.Ac. *Asian Health Secrets: The Complete Guide to Asian Herbal Medicine.* New York: Three Rivers Press, 1996.

Hobbs, Christopher. *Natural Therapy for Your Liver: Herbs and Other Natural Remedies for a Healthy Liver.* New York: Avery, a member of Penguin Putnam Inc., 2002.

Hobbs, Christopher. *Foundations of Health: Healing with Herbs and Foods.* Capitola, CA.: Botanica Press, 1992.

Hofer, Jack. *Total Massage.* New York: Grosset and Dunlap, 1976.

Horwitz, Tem, Susan Kimmelman, and H. H. Lui. *Tai Chi Ch'uan: The Technique of Power.* Chicago: Chicago Review Press, Inc., 1976.

Huang, Al Chung-Liang. *Embrace Tiger, Return to Mountain: The Essence of Tai Chi.* Moab, UT: Real People Press, 1973.

Jahnke, Roger, O.M.D. *The Healing Promise of Qi: Creating Extraordinary Wellness through Qigong and Tai Chi.* New York: Contemporary Books, 2002.

Jahnke, Roger, O.M.D. *The Healer Within.* San Francisco: HarperSanFrancisco, 1997.

Jahnke, Roger, O.M.D. *The Most Profound Medicine.* Pebble Beach, CA: Health Action Press, 1991.

Jarmey, Chris. *Taiji Qigong.* Fishbourne, Chichester, U.K.: Corpus Publishing Limited, 2001.

Jarmey, Chris, and John Tindall. *Acupressure: For Common Ailments.* New York: Simon and Schuster, 1991.

Jarret, Lonny S. *Nourishing Destiny: The Inner Tradition of Chinese Medicine.* Stockbridge, MA: Spirit Path Press, 1998.

Johnson, Larry, O.M.D., L.Ac. *Strategies: Taoist Chi Kung—Levels 1.* Crestone, CO: White Elephant Monastery, 2001.

Johnson, Larry, O.M.D., L.Ac. *Strategies: Taoist Chi Kung—Levels 2 & 3.* Crestone, CO: White Elephant Monastery, 2002.

Johnson, Larry, O.M.D., L.Ac. *Qigong.* Crestone, CO: White Elephant Monastery, 1998.

Johnson, Larry, O.M.D., L.Ac. *Qigong: A Medical I Ching Exploration.* Crestone, CO: White Elephant Monastery, 1999.

Johnson, Yanling Lee. *A Woman's Qigong Guide: Empowerment through Movement, Diet, and Herbs.* Boston: YMAA Publication Center, 2001.

Jou, Tsung Hwa. *The Tao of Meditation: Way to Enlightenment.* Boston: Charles E. Tuttle Co., 1991.

Jwing-Ming, Yang. *Qigong: The Secret of Youth: An Advanced Qigong Regimen for the Serious Practitioner.* Boston: YMAA Publication Center, 2000.

Jwing-Ming, Yang. *Qigong for Health and Martial Arts: Exercises and Meditation.* Boston: YMAA Publication Center, 1991.

Jwing-Ming, Yang. *The Essence of Tai Chi, Chi Kung: Health and Martial Arts.* Jamaica Plain, MA: YMAA Publication Center, 1990.

Kaptchuk, Ted J., O.M.D. *The Web that Has No Weaver: Understanding Chinese Medicine.* Chicago: NTC/ Contemporary Publishing Group, Inc., 2000.

Klein, Bob. *Movements of Magic: The Spirit of T'ai-Chi-Ch'uan.* Douglas Menville, ed. North Hollywood, CA: Newcastle Publishing Co., Inc., 1984.

Lade, Arnie. *Images and Functions.* Seattle: Eastland Press, 1989.

Larre, Claude, and Elisabeth Rochat de la Vallee, trans. *Rooted in Spirit: The Heart of Chinese Medicine.* New York: Station Hill Press, 1995.

Laux, Marcus, N.D., and Christine Conrad. *Natural Woman, Natural Menopause.* New York: HarperCollins Publishers, Inc., 1997.

Liang, Shou-Yu, and Wen-Ching Wu. *Qigong Empowerment: A Guide to Medical, Taoist, Buddhist and Wushu Energy Cultivation.* Denise Breiter-Wu, ed. Providence, RI: The Way of the Dragon Publishing, 1997.

Liang, Master T.T. *T'ai Chi Ch'uan: For Health and Self-Defense.* Paul B. Gallagher, ed. New York: Vintage Books, 1974.

Lidell, Lucinda, Sara Thomas, and Carol Beresford-Cooke. *The Book of Massage: The Complete Step-by-Step Guide to Eastern and Western Techniques.* New York: Simon and Schuster, 1984.

Lien-Ying, Kuo. *Tai-Chi Chuan: in Theory and Practice.* Berkeley, CA: North Atlantic Books, 1999.

Lien-Ying, Kuo, compiled and explained by. The *T'ai Chi Boxing Chronicle.* Guttman, trans. Berkeley, CA: North Atlantic Books, 1994.

Liu, Da. *The Tao of Health and Longevity.* New York: Schocken Books, 1978.

Liu, Da. *Taoist Health Exercise Book.* New York: Links Books, 1974.

Liu, Master Hong, and Paul Perry. *The Healing Art of Qi Gong.* New York: Warner Books, Inc., 1997.

Love, Dr. Susan. *Hormone Book: Making Informed Choices about Menopause.* New York: Times Books, 1997.

Love, Dr. Susan. *Breast Book.* Second edition. Reading, MA: Perseus Books, 1995.

Low, Royston. *Acupuncture in Gynaecology and Obstetrics.* Northamptonshire, England: Thorsons Publishers Ltd., 1990.

Low, Royston. *The Secondary Vessels of Acupuncture.* Northamptonshire, England: Thorsons Publishers Inc., 1983.

Lu, Nan, O.M.D., L.Ac. *A Woman's Guide to Healing from Breast Cancer: Traditional Chinese Medicine.* New York: Avon Books, 1999.

Maciocia, Giovanni. *Obstetrics and Gynecology in Chinese Medicine.* New York: Churchill Livingstone, 1998.

Maciocia, Giovanni. *The Foundations of Chinese Medicine: A Comprehensive Text for Acupuncturists and Herbalists.* New York: Churchill Livingstone, 1989.

MacRitchie, James. *Chi Kung: Energy for Life.* London: HarperCollins Publishers, 2002.

Maisel, Edward. *Tai Chi for Health.* New York: Dell Publishing., Inc., 1963.

Man-ch'ing, Cheng, and Robert W. Smith. *T'ai-Chi: The "Supreme Ultimate" Exercise for Health, Sport, and Self-defense.* Rutland, VT.: Charles E. Tuttle Co., 1967.

Masunaga, Shizuto. *Zen Imagery Exercises: Meridian Exercises for Wholesome Living.* New York: Japan Publications, 1987.

Matsumoto, Kiiko, and Stephen Birch. *Hara Diagnosis: Reflections on the Sea.* Brookline, MA: Paradigm Publications, 1988.

Matsumoto, Kiiko, and Stephen Birch. *Extraordinary Vessels.* Brookline, MA: Paradigm Publications, 1986.

Mayer, Michael. *Body, Mind, Qigong: A Training Manual of Methods and Healing Secrets.* Berkeley, CA: The Bodymind Healing Center, 1999.

McGee, Charles T., and Qigong Master Effie Poy Yew Chow. *Miracle Healing from China: Qigong.* Coeur d'Alene, ID: Medipress, 1996.

Minick, Michael. *The Kung Fu Exercise Book: Health Secrets of Ancient China.* New York: Simon and Schuster, 1974.

Namikoshi, Toru. *Shiatsu Therapy: Theory and Practice.* Tokyo: Japan Publications Inc., 1974.

Nelson, Miriam E., Ph.D. *Strong Women, Strong Bones: Everything You Need to Know to Prevent, Treat, and Beat Osteoporosis.* New York: The Berkley Publishing Group, 2000.

Ni, Maoshing, Ph.D., C.A., and Cathy McNease, B.S., M.H. *The Tao of Nutrition.* Malibu, CA: The Shrine of the Eternal Breath of Tao, 1987.

Northrup, Christiane, M.D. *The Wisdom of Menopause: Creating Physical and Emotional Health and Healing During the Change.* New York: Bantam Books, 2001.

O'Connor, John, and Dan Bensky, trans. and eds. *Acupuncture: A Comprehensive Text.* Chicago: Eastland Press, 1981.

Pike, Geoff. *The Power of Ch'i: The Secrets of Oriental Breathing for Health and Longevity.* New York: Bell Publishing Company, 1980.

Pitchford, Paul. *Healing with Whole Foods: Asian Traditions and Modern Nutrition.* Third edition. Berkeley, CA: North Atlantic Books, 2002.

Po, Li and Ananda. *Wave Hands Like Clouds: Training Method of Tai Chi.* New York: Harper and Row Publishers Inc., 1975.

Reid, Daniel. *Harnessing the Power of the Universe: A Complete Guide to the Principles and Practice of Chi-Gung.* Boston: Shambala Publications, Inc., 1998.

Requena, Yves. *Chi Kung: The Chinese Art of Mastering Energy.* Rochester, VT: Healing Arts Press, 1995.

Rolf, Ida P. *Rolfing: The Integration of Human Structures.* New York: Harper and Row Publishers, Inc., 1977.

Ross, Jeremy. *Zang Fu: The Organ Systems of Traditional Chinese Medicine.* New York: Churchill Livingstone, 1984.

Bibliography

Rubin, Alan, M.D. *Thyroid for Dummies*. New York: Hungry Minds, Inc., 2001.

Sandifer, Jon. *Acupressure: For Health, Vitality and First Aid*. Boston: Element Books, Inc., 1997.

Shanghai College of Traditional Medicine. O'Connor, John, and Dan Bensky, trans. and eds. *Acupuncture: A Comprehensive Text*. Chicago: Eastland Press, 1981.

Sivananda Yoga Center. *The Sivananda Companion to Yoga*. New York: Simon and Schuster, Inc., 1983.

Stein, Diane. *A Woman's I Ching*. Freedom, CA: The Crossing Press, 1997.

Sun, Wei Yue, M.D., and Xiao Jing Li, M.D. *Chi Kung: Increase Your Energy, Improve Your Health*. New York: Sterling Publishing Company, 1997.

Thomas, Clayton L., M.D., M.P.H, revised and edited by. *Taber's Cyclopedic Medical Dictionary,* Twelfth edition. Philadelphia: F. A. Davis Co., 1973.

Tortora, Gerard J. *Principles of Human Anatomy*. 9th edition. New York: John Wiley and Sons, Inc., 2001.

Tse, Michael. *Qigong for Health and Vitality*. Esther Jagger, ed. New York: St. Martin's Press, 1995.

Tsu, Lao. *Tao Te Ching*. Gia-Fu Feng and Jane English, trans. New York: Vintage Books, a division of Random House, 1972.

Tung, Timothy, trans. *Wushu: The Chinese Way to Family Health and Fitness*. Jane Garton, ed. New York: Simon and Schuster, 1981.

Weed, Susan S. *New Menopausal Years: The Wise Woman Way*. Woodstock, NY: Ash Tree Publishing, 2002.

Wilson, Stanley D. *Qi Gong for Beginners: Eight Easy Movements for Vibrant Health*. New York: Sterling Publishing Co., 1997.

East Asian Medical Studies Society. Wiseman, Nigel, and Andrew Ellis, translated and amended by. *Fundamentals of Chinese Medicine*. Brookline, MA: Paradigm Publications, 1985.

Xiangcai, Xu. *Qigong for Treating Common Ailments*. David Shapiro, ed. Boston: YMAA Publication Center, 2000.

Yuefang, Cen, ed. *Chinese Qigong Essentials*. Beijing: New World Press, 1996.

Zand, Janet, L.Ac., O.M.D., Allan N. Spreen, M.D., C.N.C., James B. LaValle, R.P.H., N.D. *Smart Medicine for Healthier Living: A Practical A-to-Z Reference to Natural and Conventional Treatments for Adults*. New York: Avery, 1999.

Zi, Nancy. *The Art of Breathing: Six Simple Lessons to Improve Performance, Health and Well-Being.* Gail Larrick, ed. Glendale, CA: Vivi Company, 1997.

Zhejiang College of Traditional Chinese Medicine, compiled by. *A Handbook of Traditional Chinese Gynecology.* Zhang Ting-Liang, trans., Bob Flaws, ed. Boulder, CO: Blue Poppy Press, 1987.

Videos

Choy, Howard. *Qigong Feng Shui for the Body.* Videocassette. Balmain, Australia: Sydney Tai Chi & Qigong Centre, 1999.

Cohen, Ken. *Qigong Traditional Chinese Exercises for Healing Body, Mind and Spirit.* Videocassette. Boulder, CO: Sounds True, 1996.

Hallander, Sifu Jane. *I-Chuan Chi Gong.* Videocassette. San Francisco: ALC Productions, 1995.

Hallander, Sifu Jane. *I-Chuan Chi Gong: Tape #2, I-Chuan Chi Gong Meditation.* Videocassette. San Francisco: ALC Productions, 1995.

Hallander, Sifu Jane. *I-Chuan Chi Gong: Tape #3, Advanced I-Chuan Chi Gong Exercises.* Videocassette. San Francisco: ALC Productions, 1995.

Jahnke, Roger, O.M.D. *Qigong Chi Kung,* Videocassette. Santa Barbara, CA: Health Action.

Johnson, Mark. *Tai Chi for Healing featuring the Pearl of Immortality Style.* Videocassette. Tai Chi for Healing, Mill Valley, CA: 1995.

Johnson, Mark. *Tai Chi for Seniors!* Videocassette. Mill Valley, CA.

Masterworks International. *Chi Kung Series, vol.1, The Ultimate in Health Exercise. The Five Elements and The Eight Brocades of Silk.* Videocassette. London, England: A Little Spotty Dog Production, 1994.

National Qigong Association, USA. *Discovering Qigong: Featuring the Five Treasure Set:* Videocassette. Portland, OR, 2000.

Wang, Xue Zhi. *Chi Kung Five Organ Energy Breathing.* Videocassette. San Francisco: Stine Video, 1996.

Resources

Qigong for Staying Young Website

http://www.qigong4everyone.com

Shoshanna's site offers qigong resources, links, product information support for your qigong practice, qigong tidbits, and an opportunity to enhance your qigong experience.

Red Bank Acupuncture & Wellness Center

http://www.healing4u.com

Shoshanna's wellness center provides a combination of acupuncture treatments, Chinese herbal consultations, tai chi and qigong instruction, energy body consultations, and therapeutic massage sessions. This website also offers articles, a lecture schedule, testimonials, and information about practitioners.

Women Healing Women Conferences

http://www.caringwomen.com

This website provides a schedule and information about Shoshanna's "Women Healing Women" Conferences dedicated to the health and healing of women. The conferences have hosted well-known speakers such as Coretta Scott King, Richard Simmons, Christiane Northrup, and Caroline Myss and have drawn thousands of women over the past nine years.

Governmental Agencies

White House Commission on Complementary and Alternative Medicine Policy

http://www.whccamp.hhs.gov

This commission was created by former President Clinton due to public interest in and increased use of unconventional health care. Executive Order 13147 authorizing the commission was issued on March 7, 2000. The commission has since been terminated after submitting their final report.

World Health Organization

http://www.who.int

This organization, a specialized United Nations agency for health, was established in 1948. Its objective is to achieve the highest possible level of health for all people. It is governed by 197 member states through the World Health Assembly and has set specific policy about the role of acupuncture in our health system.

The National Center for Complementary and Alternative Medicine (NCCAM)

http://www.nccam.nih.gov/

As one of the twenty-seven institutes that make up the National Institute of Health (NIH), this center supports rigorous CAM research, trains researchers in CAM, and disseminates information to the public and professionals on which CAM modalities work, which do not, and why.

Alternative Press Publications

Acupuncture Today

http://www.acupuncturetoday.com

A newspaper that creates an open forum for acupuncture and Oriental medicine including articles on acupuncture's effectiveness for various symptoms, book reviews, managed care issues, practice management, and herbal medicine news.

Alternative Medicine Review

http://www.thorne.com/altmedrev

This review publishes literature, reviews, original research, editorial comment, monographs, and book reviews on alternative medicine.

Alternative Medicine

http://www.alternativemedicine.com

This magazine offers news on herbs and supplements, natural beauty products, eating well, natural household products, and research on CAM.

Medical Acupuncture

http://www.medicalacupuncture.org/aama_marf/journal/index.html

This is a journal published by the American Academy of Medical Acupuncture for physicians by physicians. It provides a list of acupuncture physicians and promotes the integration of concepts from traditional and modern forms of acupuncture with Western medical training.

Acupuncture in Medicine

http://www.medical-acupuncture.co.uk/aimintro.htm

This is an international journal published by the British Medical Acupuncture Society. It is a Western scientific and clinical journal aimed at Western-trained physicians and health professionals that provides information on meetings and courses, suppliers, and a list of resources.

Focus on Alternative and Complementary Therapies (FACT)

http://www.ex.ac.uk/FACT

This review journal presents evidence-based CAM research in an analytical and impartial manner.

Kung Fu Qigong Magazine

http://www.ezine.kungfumagazine.com/magazine/index.php

This magazine covers all of the martial arts and the full spectrum of Chinese culture. Its website offers a forum, store, calendar of events, and resources.

Oriental Medicine Journal (OMJ)

http://www.omjournal.com

This journal has articles on acupuncture, Oriental body therapy, herbal medicine, qigong, and food therapy.

Qi Journal

http://www.qi-journal.com

This journal offers information on qigong, tai chi, Chinese medicine, culture, and philosophy, feng shui, and meditation. Its website offers more of the same.

Qi Magazine

http://www.qimagazine.co.uk/setup.htm

This magazine has qigong articles written by practitioners from China.

Spirituality and Health magazine

http://www.spiritualityhealth.com

This spiritual/religious-oriented magazine frequently publishes articles on qigong and acupuncture. Its website offers book reviews, e-courses, and events.

Tai Chi Magazine

http://tai-chi.com/magazine.htm

This international magazine provides information about tai chi, qigong, and other Chinese disciplines.

TCMWorld

http://www.tcmworld.org

This newspaper offers information about traditional Chinese medicine, natural healing, and internal martial arts. Its website has articles, discussion board, and links.

The Empty Vessel

http://abodetao.com

This magazine explores and disseminates information on qigong and nonreligious Taoist philosophy and practice. Its website includes sample articles and products, and other tools for living the Tao.

Redwing Book Company

http://www.redwingbooks.com

This company provides book titles and CD-ROMs on health, well-being, and complementary medicine. The website has a health practitioner directory as well.

Blue Poppy Enterprises

http://www.bluepoppy.com

This book company provides information about Chinese medicine and acupuncture with a line of clinical reference texts, patient-education books and pamphlets, and products for both the consumer and practitioner. Its website provides an online catalogue and learning program.

Internet Forums and Sites
Acupressure Information Website

http://www.acupressure.org

This website presents information about the field of acupressure.

WholeHealthMD

http://www.wholehealthmd.com

This website provides CAM information developed by a team of leading board-certified doctors and specialists. The site provides a reference library and information on food, healing centers, vitamins, and finding a practitioner.

International Forum for Acupuncture @ Yahoo groups

http://groups.yahoo.com/group/acupuncture

This is an Internet forum for discussion of ideas relating to the acupuncture experience. It is open to practitioners, patients, students, and other interested persons.

Internet Health Library (U.K.)

http://www.internethealthlibrary.com/index.htm

The U.K.'s largest CAM therapy and natural health-care resource website.

NaturalHealthWeb

http://www.naturalhealthweb.com

A comprehensive directory for natural health and alternative medicine.

Health World

http://www.healthy.net/qigong

This website offers a multitude of information and resources on qigong and tai chi.

Qiresearch International Forum for Qigong Research

http://groups.yahoo.com/group/qiresearch

This is an Internet forum for discussion of the scientific exploration of qigong or human subtle energy, and its applications in medicine and everyday lives.

World Qigong Event

World Tai Chi and Qigong Day

http://www.worldtaichiday.org

This website provides information about World Tai Chi and Qigong Day, an event that was first held in 1999, and which has been held in April every year since. It now includes more than 700 events in 52 countries and 46 U.S. cities.

World Qigong Federation

http://www.eastwestqi.com/wqf/wqf.htm

This organization is dedicated to the promotion of qigong as an effective mainstream method of healing. It fosters research, integrates qigong with Western medicine, and brings practitioners, scientists, and researchers together at its conferences, the World Congress on Qigong.

Organizations and Foundations

The Alternative Medicine Foundation

http://amfoundation.org

This organization provides education, information, and dialogue about the integration of alternative and conventional medicine. It provides resource guides for both professionals and the general public.

American Association of Naturopathic Physicians (AANP)

http://www.naturopathic.org

This is a national professional society representing licensed naturopathic physicians.

American Organization for Bodywork Therapies of Asia (AOBTA)

http://www.aobta.org

This organization represents and provides benefits to practitioners of Asian Bodywork Therapy. It also offers a practitioner referral service.

American Holistic Medical Association

http://www.holisticmedicine.org

This is an association geared toward professionals. It also provides consumer information and a holistic physicians referral list.

Association of Women Martial Arts Instructors

http://www.awmai.com

This organization provides networking, business education, and a list of schools and organizations for female martial artists.

National Women's Martial Arts Federation

http://www.nwmaf.org

This federation promotes involvement of women and girls in the martial arts. It offers training, a newsletter, certification, and a list of affiliated schools.

National Qigong (Chi Kung) Association * USA (NQA)

http://www.nqa.org

This association is dedicated to integrating qigong into all facets of our culture. It provides a teacher referral base, national and regional conferences, a newsletter, and China trips. It has a Women's Qigong Caucus as one of its many committees.

Pacific Association of Women Martial Artists (PAWMA)

http://www.pawma.org

This association supports women and girls in both the hard and soft traditions of martial arts throughout the Pacific region, sponsors seminars, tournaments, training camps, public demonstrations, and has a quarterly newsletter.

Qigong Association of America

http://www.qi.org

This association provides a qigong teacher referral base, a forum with discussion groups, information about classes, and educational trips to China.

The Qigong Institute

http://www.qigonginstitute.org

This organization promotes qigong through research and education. It provides news and scientific facts to aid researchers, writers, practitioners, and members of the Western medical community. It also offers a public-access page for locating qigong teachers and therapists, information about the institute's education and research activities, and a qigong database.

The American Association of Acupuncture and Oriental Medicine (AAAOM)

http://www.aaaom.org

This organization promotes high ethics and educational standards and a well-regulated acupressure profession to ensure the safety of the public. It offers national conferences to further Chinese medicine education.

The National Certification Commission for Acupuncture and Oriental Medicine (NCCAOM)

http://www.nccaom.org

This organization promotes nationally recognized standards of competence and safety in acupuncture and Oriental medicine for the purpose of protecting the public. It is the national licensing body for Oriental medicine.

Women's Qigong Alliance

http://www.thewqa.org

The organization welcomes women from all qigong, tai chi, and martial arts traditions. It is a growing community of women actively supporting one another as they develop and expand the vision of women in qigong.

Wu Dao Jing She International Qigong Society

http://www.wudaojingshe.com

This is an educational organization that facilitates the sharing of knowledge and experience among qigong practitioners. It aims to bring the benefits of qigong to the awareness of the general public.

Product Companies

Gaiam, Inc.

http://www.gaiam.com/retail/gai_shophome.asp

This company is a provider of information, goods, and services to customers who value the environment, a sustainable economy, healthy lifestyles, alternative health care, and personal development. Qi balls can be obtained from them.

Index

269

ABOUT THE AUTHOR

SHOSHANNA KATZMAN is the director and founder of the Red Bank Acupuncture and Wellness Center in New Jersey. Acupuncturist, tai chi and qigong professional, energy medicine practitioner, herbalist, and massage therapist, she has been involved in the field of traditional Chinese medicine for nearly thirty years. She has been a practitioner of tai chi and qigong since 1974, and has taught both since 1976.

Shoshanna is a nationally certified acupuncturist with a master in science in the field. She also earned a master's degree in sports medicine from San Francisco State University, where her research focused on how to teach tai chi and qigong more expertly from a Western scientific viewpoint. An adjunct professor in the Health and Fitness Department at Brookdale College in New Jersey, Shoshanna has also taught qigong to a wide range of students, including a day-long workshop reaching eight hundred high school students and Fitness after Fifty classes to hundreds of seniors.

She is currently the ambassador for the National Qigong Association (NQA), where she has met a wonderful qigong family and had the opportunity to learn from and share ideas with many well-known qigong professionals and enthusiasts. As ambassador, she has the job of bringing qigong to the public in the United States and abroad. She also serves as vice president of the NQA executive board and chair of the Healing Wave Task Force created to bring qigong across America.

An inspirational and educational speaker, Shoshanna has appeared on national television to promote awareness of holistic health and healing. Shoshanna is the co-author of *Feeling Light: The Holistic Solution to Permanent Weight Loss and Wellness* (Avon, 1997). A devoted wife and mother of three, she lives with her husband and children in Little Silver, New Jersey.